Paediatric Clinical Examination

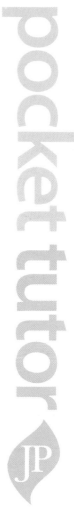

pocket tutor

Rossa Brugha BMBCh MA (Oxon) MRCPCH
Clinical Research Fellow and Honorary Specialist
Registrar in Paediatrics
Barts and the London School of Medicine and
Dentistry
London, UK

Matko Marlais BSc (Hons) MBBS (Hons)
Academic Foundation Doctor
University Hospitals Bristol NHS Foundation Trust
Bristol, UK

Ed Abrahamson MB FRCPCH
Consultant Paediatrician
Chelsea and Westminster Hospital
Honorary Senior Lecturer
Imperial College London
London, UK

JP
medical
publishers

© 2013 JP Medical Ltd.

Published by JP Medical Ltd, 83 Victoria Street, London, SW1H 0HW, UK

Tel: +44 (0)20 3170 8910 Fax: +44 (0)20 3008 6180

Email: info@jpmedpub.com Web: www.jpmedpub.com

ISBN: 978-1-907816-35-2

British Library Cataloguing in Publication Data
A catalogue record for this book is available from the British Library

Library of Congress Cataloging in Publication Data
A catalog record for this book is available from the Library of Congress

JP Medical Ltd is a subsidiary of Jaypee Brothers Medical Publishers (P) Ltd, New Delhi, India.

Publisher:	Richard Furn
Development Editor:	Paul Mayhew
Design:	Pete Wilder, Designers Collective Ltd

Indexed, typeset, printed and bound in India.

Foreword

History-taking and examination of children initially appears to be a daunting task. Children range in age from tiny newborn infants to young adults. They often do not wish to be examined, and the examiner needs to know exactly what information they are seeking and how to persuade the child to let them obtain it. Additionally, the medical conditions encountered vary markedly with age.

In *Pocket Tutor Paediatric Clinical Examination*, Rossa Brugha, Matko Marlais and Ed Abrahamson expertly guide one through dealing with these problems. As well as a brief general introduction to history and examination in children, for each system, common presentations and examination are described. This is followed by a couple of case scenarios which demonstrate how they relate to clinical practice. This information is succinctly condensed into a highly readable, pocket-sized book and is an invaluable guide to the clinical examination of children. The authors have admirably succeeded in their aim to provide a structured approach to examining children that is both stimulating and fun.

Tom Lissauer
Hon Consultant Paediatrician
Imperial College Healthcare Trust
Consultant Paediatric Programme
Director in Global Health
Imperial College London
London, UK

Preface

For those of you who have the patience and genuine passion, working with children will be one of the most rewarding and enjoyable experiences you will have in medicine. It isn't easy. Most of you reading this book will have little or no experience in managing children. *Pocket Tutor Paediatric Clinical Examination* aims to give you a structure on which to base the development of your skills. From there it's up to you. You will begin to see how flexible and adaptable you will need to be to achieve the best results, and you will develop your own style and approach.

What will also become apparent is that every case is different; each child is different, from infants from the very first minute of life, to teenagers up to 16 years of age. You will have to contend with differing abilities and levels of understanding. With this book, we aim to offer a structure that applies to all ages, but with some tweaks here and there to suit the age or particular situation you find. The book can't cover every aspect of every disease for every child. For each system, we have described a method for clinical examination alongside information about some of the common or important illnesses that you may encounter.

We hope you will find the book stimulating and fun. While occasionally we do have to deal with harrowing and exceptionally difficult situations, these are fortunately rare for most of us. For the majority of the time, paediatrics is rewarding and fulfilling. Good luck.

Rossa Brugha
Matko Marlais
Ed Abrahamson
July 2012

Contents

Chapter 15 Genetic disorders and syndromes

Acknowledgements

Thank you to Karen and Andrew Young, and their sons Jack and Daniel for kindly posing for photographs. Thank you also to Lucy Morton for photographs and for assisting with illustrations. Finally, thank you to Dr Tom Lissauer for his kind foreword.

RB, MM, EA

To my parents, and to my wife Lucy.

RB

For my wife Tanya, to whom I am eternally grateful.

MM

To my parents for getting me here, and to Stephen for his love and support in keeping me here.

EA

History taking

History-taking in paediatrics differs in many ways from history-taking in adult medicine. There are extra areas to ask about, such as perinatal history, immunisations and developmental milestones. Furthermore, babies and young children cannot speak for themselves, and history-taking becomes a three-way process involving the child, the health-care staff, and the parents or carers. Well-developed communication and perception skills are vital attributes for a paediatrician.

1.1 Algorithmic thinking

Taking a focused, or problem-oriented, history requires a higher order of thinking than a general screening history. If presenting symptoms can be immediately compared with a known list of common causes, history taking will become more effective.

Experienced doctors do algorithmic thinking without even thinking about it. It is a skill developed by seeing similar patterns over and over again. No one expects somebody who is new to paediatrics to be doing this straight away; it takes knowledge, and practice.

Clinical Scenario

A father brings an 18-month-old girl into the paediatric emergency department because she has a runny nose and is short of breath. A chest infection is a reasonable assumption. A few quick relevant questions will tease out the salient points and help to confirm or dismiss this initial hypothesis.

Consider infection – ask about fevers. No fever reported.

Reconsider – how long has she been unwell for: days? Her father says that his daughter was well until about 2 hours ago when he came back into the living room after making a cup of tea and she was suddenly very short of breath.

Reconsider – infections come on slowly, over hours or days, not minutes.

Rethink – 'sudden onset of shortness of breath in a child': the list of causes includes foreign body aspiration and pneumothorax. Eighteen-month old children put things in their mouth, and pneumothorax is uncommon in this age group. To the question, 'What was she doing?' the father replies, 'Playing with beads.' A chest X-ray shows the foreign body.

1.2 Preparation

Before entering the examination room, the doctor needs to be as well equipped as possible with key relevant information. This doesn't mean merely checking the notes for the most recent clerking; it also means collecting key information that may be important from various sources. For example, if a child is known to have a history of family neglect, particular sensitivity is required when taking a social history.

When patients are being seen in the emergency department, it is important to look at the nursing triage notes. These notes will contain useful information – for example, a brief summary of the presenting problem, and observations such as pulse rate, temperature and respiratory rate, as well as some social history. However, it is important to approach each case as new, so that (reported) previous history does not over-influence the judgement of the doctor when obtaining current information.

Setting up

Pay attention to the surroundings – this might involve pulling the curtains properly closed or shutting the door of the patient's room. Patients and parents notice these small things. A good rapport is encouraged by avoiding obstacles, such as a desk, between doctors and patients. Aim to be on a similar eye level as the child.

Children of different ages have widely varying responses to clinical situations, and they may be unaware of your presence, curious, shy, terrified, screaming, or indifferent. Each needs to be responded to appropriately; for example, an unhappy toddler who is allowed to play in a corner while the history is taken from the parents may become calmer.

1.3 Communication

The dynamics of communication in paediatrics are multilayered. Children differ in their stage of development, and there are also usually parents or other family members present, creating further challenges to a paediatrician's communication skills.

Whom am I talking to?

Most paediatric medicine involves children aged under 5 years, and therefore the history is usually taken from the parents, but this assumption is open to a number of challenges. For example, some older children have a perfectly sound appreciation of their own health (which is sometimes very different to that of the parents).

The next assumption involves the question of who is the primary carer for the child. Establish who has accompanied the child to hospital – it could be one of many people who act as carers. Do not assume that the adult who has accompanied the child is a parent.

Adults that may accompany a child include:
- parents
- grandparents, aunts and uncles
- nannies or maternity nurses
- babysitters
- teachers
- foster-parents
- social workers
- police, fire-fighters or paramedics
- neighbours
- interpreters
- figures of religious authority

There are many family units that do not fit in with the traditional family model. Be sensitive to the fact that a child may be being brought up by a same-sex couple.

Language

Check that somebody involved in the consultation speaks the same language as you, and also check what their relationship is to the patient. Interpreting is a difficult skill; be aware that interpreters who know the family may try to help by directly answering questions that are intended for somebody else. 'In your own words' is a useful phrase. Interpreters may edit your questions or the information that you give in order to protect the family, and family members may alter their answers in terms of the information they choose to give to an interpreter.

Active observation

It is useful to spend at least half the time when taking a history looking at the patient. For example, consider the 3-year-old with 'awful tummy pain' who is climbing up the chairs, as opposed to the 3-year-old with 'awful tummy pain' who is lying flat and rigid and has rapid, shallow breathing. The first is probably constipated, whereas the second probably has peritonitis.

A 1-year-old with bronchiolitis may happily sit on a parent's lap despite rapid respiration, nasal flaring, head bobbing, tracheal tug and a typical high-pitched cough. When approached, the child may start crying, preventing useful information from being gained by physical examination. Instead, therefore, sit back and observe the child for important clinical signs (explained in later chapters), many of which do not require the use of a stethoscope.

Guiding principle

The components of the paediatric history are:

- name, age, date of birth, weight
- presenting complaint
- history of the presenting complaint
- past medical history
- antenatal, birth and developmental history
- drug history (including allergies)
- immunisations
- family and social history
- systems review

1.4 Components of the paediatric history

Be sure to note:

- the name of the patient
- the age of the patient
- the date of birth of the patient
- the weight of the patient
- today's date, and the time

Presenting complaint

Start with an open question such as, 'What is the problem?' or 'How can I help?' The presenting complaint is a symptom or sign (or a collection of symptoms and signs) that have caused the parents or child to seek medical attention.

In the above example of a 1-year-old child with bronchiolitis, the presenting complaint may include one or all of difficulty breathing, cough, poor feeding and fever. The presenting complaint is the basis for forming the differential diagnosis.

History of the presenting complaint

The history should be taken as a focused, problem-based history. Aim for each question to 'rule in' or 'rule out' a possible diagnosis. Produce a summary to make sure that nothing important has been missed.

Past medical history

Enquire about previous illnesses, hospital admissions or operations.

Paediatric extras

Additionally, a paediatric history includes:
- antenatal history
- birth history
- developmental history
- immunisation history

The level of detail required depends on the context. For example, it is vital to elicit a detailed perinatal history for a child who has a developmental problem but less important for an older child with asthma.

Antenatal history

The antenatal history should cover:
- whether the pregnancy was planned or unplanned
- whether the conception was natural or, for example, by way of *in vitro* fertilisation or donor eggs
- results of antenatal ultrasound scans
- drugs used by the mother or illnesses that occurred in pregnancy
- the mother's blood group

Birth history

Make a note of:
- the type of delivery – was it spontaneous, induced, instrumental or Caesarean?
- the reasons for a Caesarean delivery

- any complications surrounding the birth
- any admission to the neonatal intensive care unit
- any treatment that was required in the postnatal ward

Developmental history

Any delayed milestones should be recorded (see Chapter 5).

Drug history

The drug history should cover:

- medications and allergies
- why the child is on any medication (some medications are used for more than one condition)
- previous medications
- non-prescribed medicines and non-medicines that the child may be taking

When giving medication doses, parents often simply give a number; check if they mean, for example, milliliters or milligrams.

Immunisations

Most countries have a national schedule for immunisation. Local policies should be checked.

The immunisation schedule may begin at birth, when some children are given the BCG vaccine, depending on local policies, which in this case are usually determined by the rate of tuberculosis in the area.

In the first 6 months of life, most immunisation programmes will provide vaccinations against diphtheria, tetanus, pertussis, *Haemophilus influenzae* type B and polio. Pneumococcal and meningococcal vaccines are also given in many countries. Hepatitis B vaccination may be offered in areas of high prevalence. At around 1 year of age, a combined mumps, measles and rubella (MMR) vaccine is widely offered. Varicella vaccination is offered in some countries but not in others (e.g. it is routine in the USA but not in the UK). There is a booster programme in the second year of life and before school age, again depending on the country.

A newer vaccine is now offered in some countries to adolescent females against the human papilloma virus, the cause of cervical cancer. This vaccination programme may be extended to adolescent males in the future.

Controversies

The past few decades have seen parents receive different and often conflicting advice on immunisations from a variety of sources, with some authors reporting serious adverse effects – such as a link between the MMR vaccine and autism, although no such link has ever been demonstrated. It is important to be able to have an informed discussion with children, parents and families about immunisation.

Family history

The doctor should ask about any major illnesses in the family, especially in children and young adults, and should also elicit if there is a history of recurrent miscarriages in the mother. This may suggest a problem with maternal health that can affect the fetus, such as systemic lupus erythematosus. Mothers who are carriers of X-linked disorders may suffer recurrent miscarriages because the disorder may be lethal to male fetuses. Ask about consanguinity in the parents.

It may be helpful to draw a family tree, going back two generations. The symbols used are shown in **Figure 1.1**. There are two reasons for doing this: either to trace a genetic illness

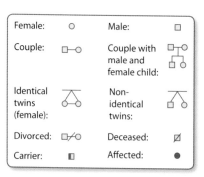

Figure 1.1 Symbols used when constructing a family tree.

through the family to establish heritability, or to work out who is who in a complex social setting.

Social history

The separation between family history and social history is rather a semantic one in paediatrics, because the family is usually the core social unit, so a family history and a social history usually overlap. A good opening question is to ask, 'Who lives at home?' Ask about school, nursery, child care and relationships, including whether the child's parents are still in a relationship with each other.

> ### Clinical insight
>
> History-taking is a dynamic process and can be revisited at any point. If awkward or difficult topics come up they can be identified for discussion later on.

Systems review

Systems review questions are particularly important when taking a history from a child with complex needs, whether the problems are neurological, developmental or associated with a syndrome. Simple, quick questions about feeding, bladder and bowels can result in valuable information if a child has, for example, cerebral palsy with severe reflux, constipation and recurrent urinary tract infections.

> ### Clinical insight
>
> **Forming a differential diagnosis**
>
> A differential diagnosis is a form of hypothesis testing. The history plus the examination findings (discussed in subsequent chapters) should lead the doctor's mind down algorithms to the point where two or three possible diagnoses are chosen. At this point, investigations may be appropriate and treatment decisions may be made.

Summary and questions

Summarise what is going on. If the child or the family feels that something has been missed, this gives a chance to go back over their concerns.

Follow this summary by giving the opportunity to ask questions. People may not ask direct questions unless they are invited to. Think about which people or agencies might have further information about the child.

Getting further information

After taking a history, think about what other sources of information may help. These may include:

- medical notes
- previous emergency department notes
- nursing staff
- discharge summaries
- the family doctor
- a community paediatrician
- previous hospitals visited
- a MedicAlert bracelet
- the school or nursery that the child attends
- health visitors
- social services
- the police

Clinical insight

Key points from this chapter:

- when asking a question while taking a history, consider how it helps to include or exclude the possibilities raised by the presenting complaint
- be quiet and listen

Examination

The point of the examination is to elicit objective information – clinical signs. The focused history should have already given clues as to what may be wrong with the child. The signs may confirm or refute this assessment, and so enable the list of possible differential diagnoses to be narrowed.

In paediatrics, there is often a mismatch between the severity of the symptoms and the clinical assessment. Therefore the examination should start at the moment the history taking begins. This can be achieved by watching the child for any worrying signs that suggest that urgent intervention may be needed.

2.1 Recognising the sick child

It may be difficult to recognise when a child is sick. Children are able to maintain their blood pressure through physiological compensation mechanisms in the early phases of serious illness, and the early signs of illness may be quite subtle. It is crucial that these early signs are detected and acted upon to prevent the child from deteriorating to the point where resuscitation is required. Once a child decompensates, he or she can collapse extremely quickly.

Clinical scenario

A mother brings her 9-month-old son to the emergency department because he has had some diarrhoea for 24 hours. His parents have not been too worried but have nevertheless decided to have the baby checked. At the start of the history-taking, however, the doctor notices that the infant appears to be pale, floppy and sleepy in his mother's arms. The doctor immediately stops taking the history and examines the child. He is very pale, has a marked tachycardia and prolonged capillary refill time (this is tested by pressing over the sternum for 3 seconds, then releasing and looking for the skin colour to return, which should take no more than 2 seconds). This child is shocked, most probably from fluid lost in the stool, and urgent resuscitation is needed. The doctor starts this while someone else continues to take the full history.

A further difficulty for inexperienced staff who assess the acutely unwell child is that children have different physiological normal values from those of adults, and inexperienced staff may be overly concerned by normal values or falsely reassured by thinking an abnormally fast pulse or a low blood pressure is normal for the child's age. See **Table 2.1** for an overview of abnormal physiological values at different ages.

Red flags

A red-flag symptom or sign (so called because a red flag indicates danger) is one that must be taken seriously and managed with the advice of senior medical and nursing staff. In paediatrics, red flags include:

- a non-blanching rash
- cool peripheries
- prolonged capillary refill
- decreased consciousness or coma
- anuria
- seizures
- haemorrhage
- a slow respiratory rate
- bradycardia
- hypotension

Clinical insight

Recognising a sick child is difficult for two main reasons:

- children are usually physically healthy and are able to compensate for illness until late in the process; then they decompensate quickly
- physiological parameters that are normal in one age group are very abnormal in another age group (see **Table 2.1**)

Age	Pulse (beats/min)	Systolic blood pressure (mmHg)	Respiratory rate (breaths/min)
0–3 months	>150	<70	>60
3–12 months	>140	<80	>50
1–5 years	>120	<85	>40
5–10 years	>110	<90	>30
>10 years	>100	<90	>25

Table 2.1 Pulse, systolic blood pressure and respiratory rate: when to be concerned about these physiological parameters, according to age

2.2 Examining a child

Ideally, when examining a child, there should be:
- a warm and clean environment
- toys and games available
- stethoscope, otoscope and tongue depressor at hand
- someone to help – a nurse or play specialist
- patience and flexibility

Environment and equipment

Aim to create an environment in which a child feels safe (**Figure 2.1**). Toys, books, television and videos or DVDs, and computer games consoles are all routine equipment in paediatric outpatient departments in many countries. Consider the micro- and macroenvironment; for example, examine a younger children on their parent's lap while they are cuddling

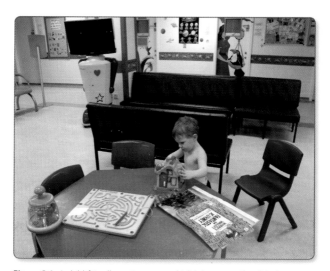

Figure 2.1 A child-friendly environment, which is important for clinical examinations.

their favourite blanket, in a warm room without draughts so that the child is comfortable when undressed.

The equipment required is:

- warm clean hands
- a smile
- a stethoscope
- a tongue depressor
- an otoscope

More specialist equipment (e.g. a tendon hammer, an ophthalmoscope) should be available nearby.

Nurses and play specialists

Nursing staff can be invaluable for distracting children during examination, and nurses may act as chaperones when older children are being examined. Play specialists are qualified in using play therapy and can distract and comfort children of all ages during painful procedures such as venesection.

Flexibility, adaptiveness, intelligence

The only firm rule when examining children is not to hurt them. Trainees examining children are not expected to follow a rigid pattern of steps. There is no need to start with the hands, as in a textbook adult examination; rather, start with what is important or what can be done, and work from there. Be practical and be adaptive – for example, if the child has erythema nodosum (a sign of inflammatory bowel disease) then check the mouth (for aphthous ulcers) and the hands (for koilonychia).

There is no need to examine the throat (an unpleasant experience for a child) if the possibility of finding useful information by examining the throat (the pre-test probability) is low.

Try to examine children in an age-appropriate way, which is often best done through mimicry. Get down to their level – on the knees if examining small children – or even below them while they are on a parent's lap (**Figure 2.2**). Similarly, when examining an adolescent, adopt the attitude that would be suitable for a young adult; doctors who unwittingly patronise adolescents and talk down to them in a babyish voice are unlikely to build good therapeutic relationships with them.

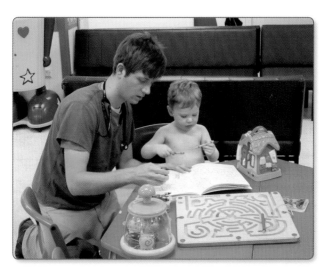

Figure 2.2 Getting down to the child's level.

Cultural considerations

Patients from cultural backgrounds that are different from your own may have different expectations from yours about the doctor–patient relationship, in terms, for example, of the sex of the examining physician or of how invasive they expect an examination to be. What may be normal or acceptable to one group of people may be abnormal to another group, and a doctor should be aware of what is considered normal to whomever he or she is looking after. This is especially important if a genital examination is required.

Crying and tantrums

Examining the crying baby

A baby that is persistently crying is a sign in itself – is it due to irritability? Alternatively, it could be due to tiredness, hunger, a need for a nappy change, colic or abdominal pain. A baby should settle when comforted by a parent or with a pacifier or a feed. This provides an opportunity to listen to the heart and breath sounds. If parents are not around, a nurse can console the baby, or a sugary solution for the baby to suck on can be tried. If the baby remains unhappy, think whether this is a sign of illness, and if in doubt, ask a more senior clinician.

Examining the unhappy toddler

A combative 2-year-old who refuses to stay on a parent's lap and runs around the room having a tantrum constitutes a good clinical sign. Children with a high fever or pain are quiet or appear unwell. Similar considerations apply to children with injuries – children with a significant head injury or a fractured limb are usually quiet and hold themselves, or the injured area, quite still. However, children may be distressed as a result of pain and this should also be considered.

If a toddler (a 1- to 3-year-old) is upset and unwilling to be examined, try another approach. Turn the child's attention by pretending to examine his or her teddy bear or a sibling; this may attract interest and the patient may come back. A firm hug from a parent, chest-to-chest, can allow access so that the back can be listened to and the abdomen palpated, and it can allow the doctor to work the stethoscope round to the front to auscultate heart sounds; it is also a good position to examine for cervical lymphadenopathy (**Figure 2.3**).

2.3 Chaperones

Clinical insight
Key points from this chapter:
• examination serves to 'rule in' or 'rule out' possible diagnoses
• it can be difficult to spot a sick child
• be considerate and flexible when examining a child, and get help if needed

It is important not to place yourself at risk when performing intimate examinations of a child. You should not perform any examination of the genitalia in any age, or the breasts when they have developed, unless a chaperone is present. The presence of a parent is not adequate.

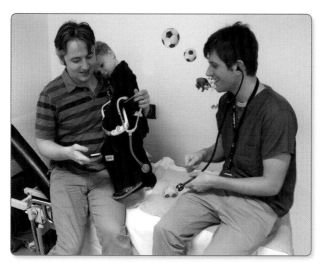

Figure 2.3 An unhappy toddler can be examined when chest-to-chest with a parent, using toys and telephones as distraction. With the child in this position it is easier to listen to the chest and feel for cervical lymph nodes.

Examination of the newborn

The key examinations of neonates are generally performed in the first few days and then at 6 weeks of age.

The baby check

Every newborn infant should undergo a routine examination in the first few days of life. This is a screening process to look for congenital conditions and to ensure normal adaptation from fetal life. The baby check is also called the neonatal examination (a neonate is defined as a newborn infant up to 28 days after their estimated delivery due date).

The 6-week check

The examination is usually repeated between 6 and 8 weeks of age to ensure that there are no new problems and that the child is growing and feeding well. In addition, there are some important problems that may not have been apparent in the first few days of life for physiological reasons, such as the murmur of a left-to-right shunt due to a ventricular septal defect (see Chapter 7).

The structure described here allows for a complete assessment of any congenital or adaptive problems and will also identify infants at particular risk of some important neonatal problems, such as sepsis.

3.1 Maternal history

Check for all maternal factors which can cause illness in the neonate (**Table 3.1**).

Maternal health before pregnancy

Maternal disorders that were present before the pregnancy commenced may affect the fetus (e.g. infections such as HIV, inflammatory disorders such as systemic lupus erythematosus).

Condition in the mother	Effects on the baby
Diabetes mellitus	Macrosomia, hypoglycaemia, polycythaemia
Hyperthyroidism	Hypothyroidism or hyperthyroidism
Systemic lupus erythematosus	Congenital heart block
Congenital infections	Microcephaly, deafness
Teratogenic medications	Spina bifida, phocomelia
Pre-eclampsia	Intrauterine growth restriction
Smoking	Decreased birth weight
Excess alcohol intake	Fetal alcohol syndrome

Table 3.1 Medical conditions in pregnancy and their effects in the newborn

Maternal health during pregnancy

Some maternal disorders develop as a direct consequence of pregnancy (e.g. gestational diabetes, pre-eclampsia). These disorders can also affect the fetus (see **Table 3.1**).

Infections during pregnancy

Furthermore, a number of acquired maternal infections are well known to cause significant morbidity and mortality in the fetus (e.g. toxoplasmosis, cytomegalovirus).

Medications and drugs

Medications or other substances taken by the mother can seriously affect the infant; for example:
- lithium (a mood stabiliser) can cause cardiac abnormalities
- smoking decreases the fetal birth weight
- excessive intake of alcohol may result in the fetal alcohol syndrome, which is characterised by dysmorphic features and impaired intelligence

The neonatal examination should commence with a check of the maternal notes for all of these factors, including the results of any screening investigations such as HIV and hepatitis B serology and the results of any blood tests to look for any risk of underlying chromosomal abnormalities in the infant.

3.2 History relating to the fetus

Fetal health

In addition to checking the maternal factors discussed above, check to see if there were any concerns relating to the health of the fetus, such as threatened miscarriage, poor growth or breech position.

Look at the reports of the antenatal scans – were any abnormalities identified? Check to see if any genetic testing was carried out on the fetus, such as amniocentesis or chorionic villus sampling, and if so what the results were.

Look at the expected due date and calculate the baby's gestation. Term is 37–42 weeks.

Labour and delivery

Check the labour and birth notes to see if there was any evidence of fetal distress, such as an abnormal cardiotocography tracing or meconium-stained liquor (a stressed infant may open the bowels and pass meconium). Also check whether the delivery was normal vaginal, instrumental or Caesarean.

Check whether any resuscitation of the newborn was required following birth.

Look at the Apgar score (**Table 3.2**). This score is calculated at 1 minute, 5 minutes and 10 minutes after birth. An Apgar score of less than 2 at 5 minutes after delivery correlates with a higher risk of long term problems with neurological development.

Plot the birth weight on the appropriate chart.

See if there are any risk factors for sepsis in the baby.

> ## Clinical insight
>
> Risk factors for sepsis in newborn babies include:
> - premature labour (earlier than 37 weeks' gestation)
> - prolonged rupture of membranes (>24 hours)
> - maternal group B Streptococcus colonisation (on vaginal swab)
> - maternal fever during labour

Score	0	1	2
Colour	White	Blue	Pink
Tone	None, floppy	Some flexion	Actively flexed
Breathing	Not breathing	Weak, irregular, gasps	Good cry or regular respirations
Heart rate	No heart rate	<100 beats/min	>100 beats/min
Response to stimulation	No response	Weak grimace or feeble cry	Good cry, flexed tone

Table 3.2 Apgar score. Calculate the total by scoring the baby for each feature. Aggregate the scores to reach a total (maximum 10).

3.3 Examination of the newborn

Start the examination by taking the opportunity to talk to the baby's mother about how the pregnancy and delivery were, and how she feels her baby is. While doing this, observe the baby and look around the bed looking for any clues – bottle milk and discarded nappies can give information about feeding and about whether the baby has opened their bowels.

Enquire about breast-feeding, and encourage it if appropriate.

Ask whether the baby has passed urine and meconium (the first stools passed by a baby). Babies should open their bowels within the first 24 hours of life.

Clinical insight

If the baby is asleep, it is advisable to listen to the heart sounds before undressing the baby and causing crying. If the baby is already unsettled, go through the rest of the examination in a systematic manner and try to settle the baby later on for the cardiac examination.

General inspection
Colour

Check the baby's colour to ensure that the baby is not cyanosed (suggestive of a severe cardiac or respiratory disorder) or grey (suggestive of a cardiac disorder or sepsis).

Appearance

Does the baby look dysmorphic (an abnormal facial appearance suggestive of a genetic abnormality)? In the first few days the face may appear swollen, with bruising caused by the delivery; if this is the case, wait a further 24 hours to make a judgement.

If the child is awake, observe the muscle tone and movements (**Figure 3.1**).

Skull

When examining the skull, the following should be looked for:

- overlapping sutures

Clinical insight

When a baby check is being done, the following should be examined:

- general appearance – is the baby well or unwell?
- tone and posture
- colour
- skull and head circumference
- ears, eyes, nose and mouth
- skin
- shoulders, arms and hands
- chest and heart sounds
- abdomen
- groin
- genitalia
- femoral pulses
- legs and feet
- spine
- reflexes
- hips

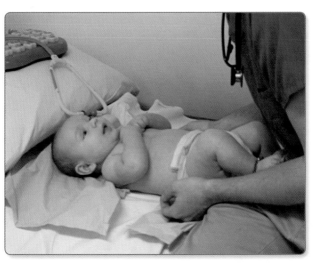

Figure 3.1 General inspection: normal flexed tone in a neonate.

- the caput (checking for moulding)
- cephalhaematoma (bleeding between the skull bone and periosteum)
- subgaleal bleed (bleeding between the periosteum and the aponeurosis)

Measure and plot the occipitofrontal head circumference. This measurement is made by placing a measuring tape around the head, and measuring the circumference that includes both the forehead and the occiput (**Figure 3.2**).

Ears

Look for pits (small holes) and tags (small protrusions of extra skin) anterior to the tragus. Babies with pits may have abnormal inner ear architecture and therefore need extra hearing screening.

Eyes

Observe the eye movements and elicit the red reflex in each eye. This is done by looking into the eye through the ophthalmo-

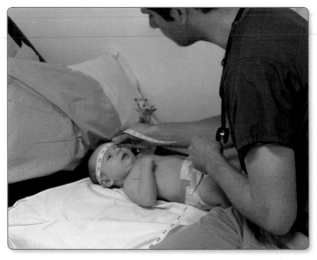

Figure 3.2 Measuring the occipitofrontal circumference.

scope from a distance and seeing the red reflection of the retina (much like when using a flash on a camera and seeing a 'red eye' reflection). With a normal reflex the back of the eye, the retina, appears a healthy pink or red colour.

The presence of a normal retinal light reflection rules out a congenital cataract. A child with leukocoria, in which the pupil appears white, may have a cataract and should be referred urgently to an ophthalmologist.

Nose and mouth

Inspect the nose and mouth to check for patent nares or a choanal atresia (in which one or both nostrils are occluded by bone). Babies are obligate nasal breathers and therefore a blocked nostril is an important finding – a baby with a blocked nostril may be stressed by feeding.

Inspect and palpate inside the mouth for cleft lip or cleft palate, and check the sucking (or 'rooting') reflex by placing a finger inside the mouth (**Figure 3.3**). Check for the presence

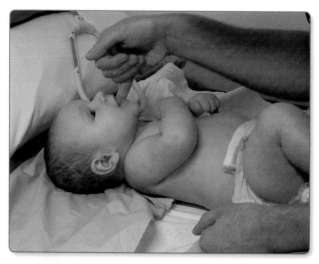

Figure 3.3 The sucking reflex. The baby turns the head to the side if the cheek is rubbed and searches for a nipple ('rooting'), then sucks strongly in a co-ordinated fashion.

of teeth. Babies may be born with teeth, and these are often loose. Teeth should be removed because they pose a risk of aspiration and can impair breast-feeding.

Skin

There are numerous benign neonatal skin conditions, of which erythema toxicum is the commonest. A small, raised white spot is surrounded by a 1–2 mm ring of erythema. The spots may become confluent, resulting in an impressive rash all over the trunk with numerous white spots; however, the baby is otherwise completely well. In this situation, the parents can be reassured.

Clavicles

The clavicle may be fractured during an obstructed labour. Palpate along the length of the bone for any crepitus or swelling.

Arms

Observe the arms for Erb palsy and Klumpke palsy. These conditions are caused by trauma to the brachial plexus during passage through the birth canal:

- in Erb palsy (in which the superior nerve roots have been affected), the child holds the affected arm extended with the wrist flexed (the 'waiter's tip' posture)
- in Klumpke palsy, the opposite occurs – the inferior nerve roots are affected and the arm is held flexed across the body

Hands

Look at the number of palmar creases. A single palmar crease may be seen in Down syndrome (trisomy 21), but a single crease is also a normal variant in the population.

Check the number of digits, and look for accessory digits. These may be small and tethered to the adjacent finger by a small skin bridge. They are described as preaxial if they are on the radial side of the hand, and postaxial if they are on the ulnar side (attached to the little finger).

Assess for abnormalities of the fingers, looking for small curved fingers (clinodactyly) and for fingers that remain fused together (syndactyly).

Check the grasp reflex (**Figure 3.4**).

Chest

Look at the shape of the chest. Both pectus carinatum ('pigeon chest') and pectus excavatum (a 'hollow' chest shape with a deeply recessed sternum) can cause problems with respiration.

Count the respiratory rate, and observe the baby for signs of respiratory distress (see Chapter 6). An unwell neonate often displays signs of respiratory distress; for example, respiratory distress may occur in a baby with sepsis, hypoglycaemia, hypercarbia or hypoxia.

Hyperplasia of the breast tissue may be observed in both male and female neonates as a result of maternal breast-stimulating hormones crossing the placenta. A small amount of milk may also be produced.

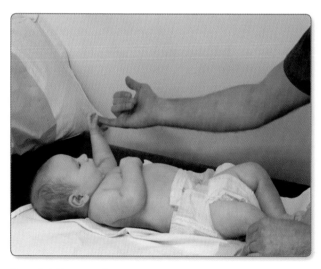

Figure 3.4 The grasp reflex.

Auscultate for respiratory sounds, checking that air entry is equal on the two sides. Pneumothorax is thought to occur in one in 100 newborns. Most of these pneumothoraces are not clinically obvious, but pneumothorax should be considered in a neonate who becomes acutely unwell with respiratory distress.

Heart

Listen to the heart sounds (**Figure 3.5**). A baby who is crying may settle on sucking a parent's finger or a pacifier. For a description of cardiac auscultation, see Chapter 7. Cardiac auscultation is a difficult skill and one that requires much practice.

Femoral pulses

Feel for the femoral pulses on both sides to assess for good-volume pulses. See **Figure 3.6** for a suggested technique for doing this. Impalpable femoral pulses are a very serious sign, because it may indicate an impending coarctation of the aorta.

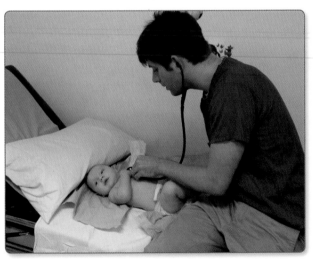

Figure 3.5 Listening to the heart sounds.

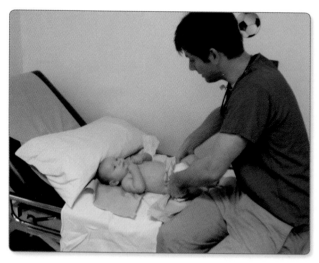

Figure 3.6 Palpating for femoral pulses. With the radial border of the index finger in the popliteal fossa, the thumb should line up in place over the femoral pulse.

Abdomen

Palpate for organomegaly (**Figure 3.7**) It is normal to feel a 1 cm liver edge, as the chest wall does not normally completely cover the liver in neonates.

Inspect the umbilical stump – it should be clean and dry. An umbilical stump or periumbilical skin that is wet, infected, malodorous or inflamed raises concerns of infection. Infection from the umbilical stump (omphalitis) can spread rapidly to the liver, which may feel 'woody' and hard and will be very tender, making the baby cry on palpation.

Groin

Inspect for hernias. An inguinal hernia in a female baby may contain the ovary. A neonate with a hernia should be referred to a paediatric surgeon.

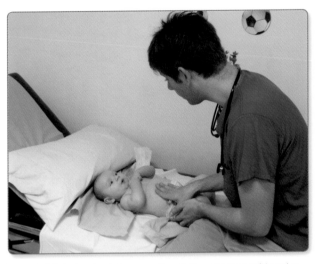

Figure 3.7 Palpating the abdomen gently, with the radial border of the index finger feeling for a liver edge that moves with respiration.

Genitalia

In males

Inspect the penis for epispadias or hypospadias; the urethral meatus may be sited on the dorsal or ventral shaft.

Palpate the testes to check that they are descended. In baby boys the testes may be retractile, i.e. they sit in the inguinal region but can easily be brought down. If a testis on one side is impalpable then an ultrasound is required to locate it.

In females

Look for normal female genitalia. The genitalia may be virilised in conditions such as congenital adrenal hyperplasia. There is often some minor bleeding per vagina in baby girls following birth – this is analogous to a withdrawal bleed, occurring when the effect of maternal progesterone on the girl's uterus during the pregnancy is lost and some endometrium is shed.

Anus

Inspect to ensure that the anus appears patent; a child may pass meconium through a fistula or the vagina, and therefore a history of opening the bowels is not enough to exclude a low rectal or anal atresia. Anal atresia is associated with Down syndrome (trisomy 21) (see Chapter 15).

Legs

Look for talipes (club foot). If it is present, assess whether it is postural (in which case the foot can be straightened) or fixed (in which case the curved shape of the foot cannot be returned to normal by stretching).

Check the number of digits, and look for any accessory digits.

Spine
Skin

Turn the baby over and inspect the back, looking again at the skin. It is common to see a blue spot (some textbooks describe this as a 'Mongolian blue spot'). This is a blue discoloration of the skin, usually across the sacrum and buttocks. It is a common congenital skin finding (or birthmark), especially in children with darker skin pigmentation. It is important to record the presence of a blue spot because it may be confused later with bruising and therefore raise concerns regarding child safety – medical notes from the neonatal check may be crucial in establishing whether a baby has been harmed. It is important that such notes are comprehensive and accurate.

Spina bifida

Look for tufts of hair or pits in the natal cleft. Pits in the natal cleft are common and are not concerning unless the base of the defect cannot be seen, in which case an ultrasound is required to ascertain whether the pit extends down to the spinal cord, where it may affect the nerve roots or communicate with the structures of the spinal cord (as in spina bifida).

True spina bifida is rare in those countries in which folate is given routinely to women during pregnancy, because such supplementation decreases the risk of neural tube defects. It remains common in countries where mothers are not able to take folate around the time of conception and during the first trimester of pregnancy.

Reflexes

Examination of the reflexes, together with the hip examination, are best left until the end of the baby check. There are a number of primitive reflexes, but the key ones to test are:

- the Moro reflex
- the stepping reflex

For a fuller explanation of reflexes in neonates and young children, see Chapter 9.

The Moro reflex

The most important reflex to elicit as part of the newborn examination is the Moro or 'startle' reflex. It is elicited by making the baby feel as if they are falling. Support the back with one hand and the head with the other (**Figure 3.8**), and then bring

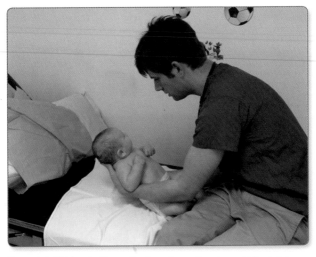

Figure 3.8 Eliciting the Moro reflex. From the position shown, let the baby's head fall back gently by 2–3 cm; the baby will fling out the arms in a 'startle' or Moro reflex.

both hands down quickly approximately 2 or 3 cm so the baby momentarily falls backwards – at this point the baby will throw both arms out symmetrically in abduction and then bring the forearms together towards the midline.

A normal Moro reflex implies that there are intact neuro-muscular connections from the central nervous system to the muscles in the upper limbs. The Moro reflex may be absent on one side if there is damage to the peripheral nerves on that side (as may occur in a brachial plexus injury during birth). In hypoxic ischaemic encephalopathy secondary to a lack of oxygen during labour, the Moro reflex may be either very pronounced (with the baby startling to minimal stimulation) or, in severe encephalopathy, absent.

The stepping reflex

The stepping reflex (**Figure 3.9**) demonstrates normal neural connections to the legs. Hold the baby in a standing position and slowly move the baby forwards with the toes touching the

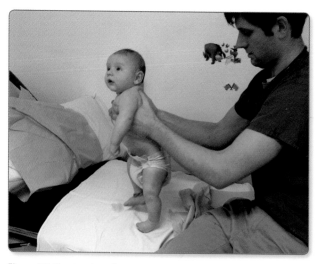

Figure 3.9 The stepping reflex.

bed – the baby will lift the feet and place them in front of each other, as if walking.

The feet also have a grasp reflex (**Figure 3.10**). To elicit this, stroke the sole of the foot – the toes will curl to grasp the object.

Hips

Examination of the hips often causes a baby to cry, and it is therefore best left until last. The examination aims to determine whether the baby has developmental dysplasia of the hip, in which the acetabulum is too shallow and the hip can be dislocated. There are two tests, the Barlow test and the Ortolani test.

The Barlow test

The Barlow test (**Figure 3.11**) examines whether the head of the femur is in place but can be dislocated posteriorly. This can be remembered as **B**arlow = **b**ack.

The technique involves pushing the femur posteriorly (backwards). With the baby lying supine, adduct the hip so that the knees are touching in the midline with the knees flexed at 90°.

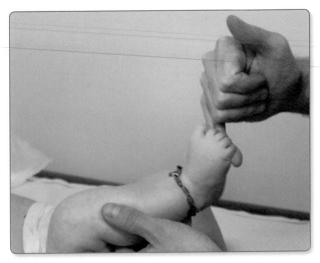

Figure 3.10 The grasp reflex in the foot.

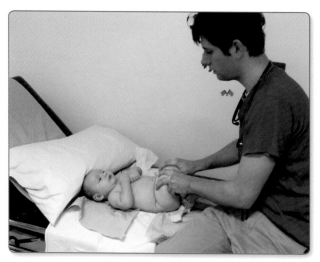

Figure 3.11 The Barlow test. Try to see if the hip will dislocate posteriorly by pushing the femur backwards, out of the acetabulum.

With an index finger on the greater trochanter of each femur, push the knees backwards in an attempt to dislocate the hip posteriorly. If the hip does dislocate, there may be a palpable 'clunk'. Examine each leg in turn.

The Ortolani test

The Ortolani test (**Figure 3.12**) aims to relocate a hip that is already dislocated. This can be remembered as **O**rtolani = **o**pen. With the baby's knees flexed at 90° and touching each other, place an index finger on the greater trochanter and externally rotate the femurs, opening up the legs. If the head of the femur is posteriorly dislocated this will relocate the joint, and there will be a 'clunk' as the head of the femur pops back into the acetabulum. Again, examine each leg in turn.

Finishing the examination

Finish the neonatal check by offering to dress the baby and address any questions. Wash your hands.

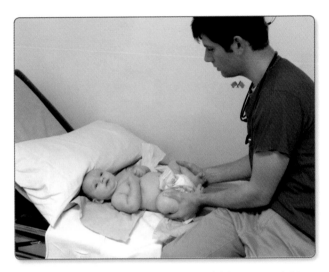

Figure 3.12 The Ortolani test. Try to see if the hip will dislocate anteriorly. Bring the head of the femur forwards out of the acetabulum by palpating the greater trochanter and opening out the hips.

3.4 Clinical scenario

A neonate with a rash

A midwife is concerned about a rash on a newborn baby; the mother has brought the rash to her attention and the midwife would like another person to look at it. The baby seems well, although there is an extensive rash on the trunk and back. There are multiple small pustules with small red halos around them. Because the child is well and the appearance of the rash is typical of erythema toxicum, you are happy to reassure the mother that the rash will disappear within a week or two.

The mother states that she is also worried about the child's hips, because she herself had an operation on her hips when she was a child. She knows that hip problems can run in families: her older child was screened. A baby check examination shows that the left hip is positive to the Ortolani test, and this is subsequently confirmed by a senior colleague. An ultrasound shows a shallow acetabulum, and the baby is referred to the orthopaedic team for splints and follow-up.

Clinical insight

Key points from this chapter:
- the baby check is a screening tool for congenital abnormalities
- know the routine and cover all parts of the examination from head to toe

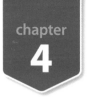

Growth and nutrition

Adequate nutrition is fundamental to normal growth and development in infants and children. There are many adverse health consequences of a diet that either lacks calories and micronutrients (poor weight gain, recurrent infections, rickets, scurvy) or that offers excessive calories (obesity, diabetes).

Growth and energy

The period of greatest growth is during the first year of life; children generally triple their birth weight by 12 months of age. They have a very high energy requirement, some three times that of an adult (150 ml/kg/day of milk, approximately 100 kcals/kg/day). **Table 4.1** shows the fluid requirements for infants.

Feeding

Newborn babies are fed exclusively on milk until weaning at 4–6 months of age, with breast milk (unless contraindicated; see **Table 4.2**) offering clear advantages over formula milk, such as a reduced risk of infection in the infant. Approximately 10% of the protein in breast milk is maternal immunoglobulin (IgA),

Age	Required intake (ml/kg/day)
Day 1	60
Day 2	90
Day 3	120
Day 4	150
Month 1	150
Month 2	120–150
Month 3 to 6	100–120

Table 4.1 Fluid requirements for infants up to 6 months of age.

| Certain maternal medications (check local formularies) |
| Maternal HIV infection* |
| Untreated maternal tuberculosis |
| Cleft lip and palate (babies can be fed maternal milk via special bottles) |

*Maternal HIV infection is a relative contraindication to breast-feeding: vertical transmission has been described, and in developed countries maternal HIV is considered a contraindication; however, if the mother and baby are in an area where water supplies may not be clean, the risk to the baby from water-borne infection may be greater than the risk of vertical transmission of HIV

Table 4.2 Contraindications to breast-feeding.

which provides immune protection to the newborn as its own immune system develops.

Vitamins and minerals

A child's diet requires adequate quantities of vitamins and minerals for normal growth. The most common vitamin deficiency is of vitamin D, caused by a combination of low vitamin D intake (e.g. prolonged breast-feeding by a mother with low vitamin D levels) and insufficient skin exposure to sunlight. If severe, vitamin D deficiency can lead to rickets, which affects the metaphyses of the bones, the site of fastest bone growth. The clinical features of this are swelling of the wrists, ankles or knees, and X-rays can show cupping and fraying of the metaphyseal region of the long bones (**Figure 4.1**).

An underlying malabsorptive state predisposes to many other vitamin deficiencies. For example, in cystic fibrosis the absorption of the fat-soluble vitamins (vitamins A, D, E and K) is impaired as a result of pancreatic insufficiency.

4.1 Common nutritional and growth problems

Common presentations related to nutrition and growth include:
- failure to gain weight in the neonatal period
- faltering weight in a 9-month-old infant
- short stature

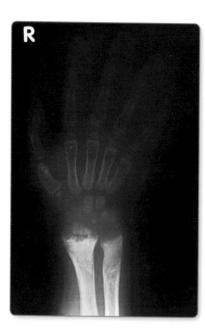

Figure 4.1 X-ray of a wrist demonstrating metaphyseal cupping and splaying caused by vitamin D deficiency.

Failure to gain weight in the neonatal period

Failure of neonatal weight gain is a common problem, and it is an important one to address. The main causes are:

- primary lactation failure (in breast-fed infants)
- milk allergy or lactose intolerance
- congenital disorders

Primary lactation failure

Breast-fed infants commonly experience some weight loss in the first 5 days of life, and it is not uncommon for it to take up to 14 days for the original birth weight to be regained. However, on occasion, weight loss is excessive (e.g. more than 10% of the birth weight) or prolonged (when birth weight has not been regained by day 14).

Clinical features The baby may be obviously thin with loose skin folds, and in severe cases the baby may become sleepy and jaundiced. The serum sodium may be increased as a result of insufficient water intake (hypernatraemic dehydration), and the blood sugar may be low because of an inadequate calorie intake (neonatal hypoglycaemia). This is a potentially dangerous situation for the infant, because there is a risk of a stroke or seizures.

Management These infants require top-up feeding by bottle at the end of every breast-feed, using either expressed breast milk, if it is available, or formula milk. Feeding by nasogastric tube may be needed in severe cases.

Milk allergy or lactose intolerance

Another cause of failure to gain weight in the neonatal period is primary lactose intolerance or an allergy to milk protein. This can occur even in breast-fed infants as maternal ingestion of milk protein can still affect the infant.

Clinical features There may be symptoms of diarrhoea, particularly in lactose intolerance, in which the stool is watery and acidic and may cause marked perianal excoriation. Other possible symptoms include abdominal pain (which manifests itself as bad colic), vomiting, discomfort on feeding, and squirming.

Management When milk allergy or lactose intolerance is suspected, it is worth the mother having a trial of avoiding all dairy products. Replacing breast milk with a specialised lactose-free or hydrolysed protein formula may also be indicated.

Congenital causes

There are numerous congenital causes of poor weight gain in the neonatal period. The main ones are listed in **Table 4.3**. The approach to this problem is complex and requires a detailed investigative approach based on the clinical appearance and the likelihood of the various possible causes.

Faltering weight in a 9-month-old infant

Faltering weight at 9 months of age is a very common clinical problem. Faltering weight is usually defined as the crossing of 2 centiles on the growth chart.

Type of problem	Example
Chromosomal disorder	Down syndrome (trisomy 21)
Metabolic disorder	Galactosaemia
Liver disease	Biliary atresia
Congenital heart disease	Ventricular septal defect
Congenital infection	Cytomegalovirus

Table 4.3 Examples of congenital causes of poor weight gain in neonates.

The causes can be broadly divided into:
- lack of intake
- excess losses (from vomiting, diarrhoea or malabsorption)
- increased metabolic demand

Lack of intake

Inadequate intake can result from:
- inadequate offered milk, e.g. lactation failure
- weaning failure
- physical barriers to feeding, e.g. cleft palate
- behavioural feeding problems

Inadequate offered milk Inadequate milk being offered can be due to lactation failure, as outlined above, and it can also occur when an infant simply requires more milk than is being offered. Although in most cases the latter is caused by an innocent underestimate of how much milk the infant requires, it can be part of child neglect, in which there is a general failure to provide for the infant's needs.

Weaning failure Most infants are weaned on to solids by 6 months of age, and as the solid diet becomes more established they will drink less and less milk. However, some infants fail to wean and remain fully milk-fed, and this can be a particular problem with infants who have been exclusively breast-fed. Both the quality and quantity of breast milk tends to lessen beyond 6 months, and it may not be adequate to meet the infant's needs after this time.

Physical barriers to feeding There are many physical problems that can affect infant feeding, and the clinical assessment must exclude all of these issues. Key causes include:

- cleft palate
- tongue tie
- abnormalities of the chin (e.g. micrognathia, as occurs in Pierre Robin sequence)
- choanal atresia, in which the nasal passages are blocked and the infant cannot breathe with the mouth closed

Behavioural feeding problems A reluctance or refusal to feed on milk or solids is common, and often follows on from an earlier period when there was an association between feeding and pain, as may occur with oesophagitis, for example. In severe cases, this problem requires the support of a feeding team that includes speech and language therapists and psychologists.

Excess losses

Losses may be obvious (e.g. from vomiting or frank diarrhoea) or less obvious (e.g. from malabsorption, in which the stools can be simply bulky and smelly).

Common causes of excess losses include:

- gastroesophageal reflux
- pyloric stenosis
- lactose intolerance
- coeliac disease
- cystic fibrosis

Increased metabolic demand

Any condition in which the child has a higher need for calories may cause poor growth.

Common causes include:

- chronic respiratory illness with tachypnoea
- congenital cardiac disease
- chronic infections, e.g. HIV
- inborn errors of metabolism – many rare disorders involve various enzyme deficiencies

Short stature

The main causes of short stature to be considered are:
- familial short stature
- constitutional delay of growth and puberty
- growth hormone deficiency
- genetic syndromes
- chronic illness, including malnutrition

Familial short stature

Clinical features A child with familial short stature will fall within the expected centile range, based on the mid-parental height (see below). The growth velocity, as measured over a minimum of 6 months, is normal.

Constitutional delay of growth and puberty

Clinical features In a child with constitutional growth delay there is no underlying abnormality, and although the child may appear to be falling off the normal growth centiles, he or she will eventually catch up once puberty commences.

A wrist X-ray can enable a bone age to be measured, and this age can be compared with the chronological age to ascertain if there is any constitutional delay.

Growth hormone deficiency

Growth hormone deficiency can be:
- idiopathic
- secondary to pituitary dysfunction, as may occur with a pituitary tumour or following irradiation

Clinical features In a child with growth hormone deficiency, growth velocity falls below the minimum (4 cm/year) that is required for normal growth. Most commonly the inadequate growth velocity is noted in mid-childhood. The child may also appear slightly overweight.

Measurement of growth velocity is required over a 6-month period. If it is found to be reduced, formal investigations should be undertaken to confirm the cause. These investigations involve complex tests that are performed only in specialist centres.

Genetic syndromes

There are many syndromes associated with short stature, such as Turner syndrome and Noonan syndrome(see Chapter 15). Sometimes there will be phenotypic features that suggest an underlying syndrome, but occasionally – for example in mosaic forms – this is not so. It is generally appropriate to check a karyotype as part of the investigations for short stature.

Chronic illness

Any chronic illness, such as poorly controlled asthma, inflammatory bowel disease or malnutrition, can be associated with poor growth velocity. A full history and examination is needed to look for any evidence of underlying disease.

4.2 Examination

General assessment

Measurements of growth

Accurate measurements of height, weight and head circumference should be taken, included in the patient's notes and plotted on a growth chart. These measurements can provide diagnostic clues even before the formal clinical examination is begun – for example, they may provide information about whether the child is maintaining centiles or falling away significantly.

Head circumference is measured by placing a tape measure around the occiput and the forehead to obtain the occipito-frontal circumference (see Chapter 3).

Height should be measured with the patient's footwear removed.

A baby's weight should be measured with the baby naked; a child's weight should be measured with the child in underwear (if practical).

General inspection

Check to see if the child appears dysmorphic (which may indicate the existence of a syndrome).

Look for any loose skin folds or muscle wasting suggestive of significant malnutrition.

Look at the abdomen for distension (as may occur in malnutrition or malabsorption).

Hands and lymph nodes

Look for clubbing (which suggests various chronic illnesses) and signs of anaemia.

Cervical lymphadenopathy

Examine the cervical lymph nodes for swelling, which can suggest chronic infections.

Face

Check the sclerae for jaundice (seen in liver disease).

Examine the mouth and tongue; there may be aphthous ulcers and loose teeth in vitamin C deficiency (scurvy).

Chest and abdomen

Examine the chest for evidence of any chronic respiratory disease (see Chapter 6). Listen for heart murmurs, which may indicate congenital heart disease (see Chapter 7).

Examine the abdomen for hepatosplenomegaly, as may occur in chronic haematological disease.

Limbs

Look for evidence of rickets, such as:
- swelling around the wrists
- swelling in the costochondral junctions ('rickety rosary')
- bowing of the legs

Pubertal status

When there is concern about growth in an older child, the pubertal status should be examined. Breast development, testicular size, and pubic and axillary hair should be checked. These can be measured against centiles for normal pubertal development.

Growth parameters

Standard quantitative measurable variables that have a normal distribution – weight, height or length, and head circumference – should be plotted on to growth charts, which can then be used to compare individual measurements against data gathered from the normal population of the same age.

Most children will already have had some previous records plotted, because in many countries every child has some form of health record. Single point measurements with no previous records for comparison are of limited use.

Note any discrepancies, such as the weight being relatively much greater than the height, which may be due to obesity or to an underlying syndrome such as Prader–Willi syndrome (see Chapter 15), or the head circumference being relatively much greater than the weight, which suggests possible hydrocephalus, past meningitis or traumatic head injury.

Clinical insight

Calculating mid-parental height

For girls:

- Subtract 13 cm from the father's height, add the corrected father's height and mother's height, and divide by 2

    [(father – 13) + mother]/2 = mid-parental height

For boys:

- Add 13 cm to the mother's height, add the corrected mother's height and the father's height, and divide by 2

    [(mother + 13) + father]/2 = mid-parental height

Mid-parental height

Because the population data for height, weight and head circumference have a normal distribution, 5% of patients will, by definition, be 'outliers'. To appreciate what is normal for any given child, it is important to compare the child's biophysical profile with his or her genetic potential (i.e. the child's measurements should be interpreted in the context of a comparison with the parents' measurements, using the mid-parental height).

To calculate the mid-parental height, measure the height of both parents. If the child is a girl, convert her father's height to a female height: on average men are 13 cm taller than women, so to make this conversion, subtract 13 cm from the father's height. Now add the mother's height and the father's corrected height and divide by two, and then plot this point on the growth chart at age 18 years. Note the centile that this height gives, and compare it with the centile that the child is currently at. If the child is a boy, a similar correction is made by subtracting 13 cm from the mother's height.

This comparison with the mid-parental height can allay the anxiety of tall parents who are concerned about a tall child and of short parents who are concerned about a child's apparent slow growth.

4.3 Clinical scenario

An 18-month-old boy with poor weight gain

An 18-month-old Caucasian boy is referred to the paediatric clinic because his parents are concerned about the weight of this, their second son. He had a normal birth weight (3.7 kg; 75th centile) but at 1 year of age he weighed 8.2 kg (9th centile) and now he weighs 8.6 kg (2nd centile). He had four lower respiratory infections in his first year of life, which were thought to be recurrent bronchiolitis. The only other feature of note in the history is that his mother says that his stools are very different from those of his elder brother.

Differential diagnosis

The child has failure to thrive; he has dropped from the 75th to the 2nd centile. The following possibilities should be considered:

- inadequate nutritional intake (perhaps due to poor feeding as a result of reflux)
- malabsorption (perhaps due to allergy or to pancreatic insufficiency),
- increased losses (perhaps due to an inflamed bowel resulting from infection or due to coeliac disease)

- increased use of calories (as a result of increased muscle energy use, e.g. secondary to tachypnoea in cardiac failure)

There is no history of poor feeding. He has abnormal bowel motions so this could be a result of malabsorption. Chest infections may point to cystic fibrosis, although he may have simply had repeated viral upper respiratory tract infections. His parents are Caucasian, which increases the likelihood of both coeliac disease and cystic fibrosis, because of the higher than average carrier frequencies for these disorders in the Caucasian population.

Investigations

The plot of the boy's weights shows definite failure to thrive (i.e. the weight crossing 2 or more centiles), and the history prompts a coeliac screen and a sweat test. Sweat chloride is >100 mmol, which is positive: the diagnosis is therefore cystic fibrosis.

Developmental assessment

Assessing a child's developmental age is a difficult skill that requires a knowledge of developmental milestones and of the assessment techniques.

There are four developmental domains:

- fine motor and vision
- gross motor
- social
- speech and hearing

Children develop at different rates, and there is a wide range of variation and normality. Some children skip stages; for example, some never crawl but go straight to walking. Some children can be advanced in one area but lag behind in another and yet go on to acquire the delayed skills eventually.

5.1 Developmental milestones

The developmental milestones (**Table 5.1; Figures 5.1–5.8**) have an age limit by which they should be reached; for example, a child ought to be walking by the age of 18 months. If a milestone has not been reached by the age limit, investigations should be considered. However, any concerns over development need to be carefully managed and the child watched over time, to avoid making a wrong diagnosis and causing unnecessary parental upset. Most cases of apparent delay turn out to be 'delayed normal'.

5.2 Developmental assessment

Developmental assessment is a unique skill in medicine. Whereas clinical examination is about looking for physical signs that indicate disease, developmental assessment is about looking for abilities or actions that should be present.

Age	Fine motor and vision	Gross motor	Social skills	Speech and hearing
6 weeks	Fixes and follows, initially through 45° degrees, then 90° (see Figures 5.1 and 5.2); closed hands	Head lag on pull to sit; holds head in line on ventral suspension (see Figure 5.3)	Smiles at parent's face	Quietens in response to sound
3 months	Fixes and follows through 180°; hands open; beginning to bring hands to midline	No head lag on pull to sit (see Figure 5.4); raises head to 90° when prone	Social smiling (realises smiling makes another person smile in response) (see Figure 5.5)	Turns head to sound; coos in response
5–6 months	Voluntary grasp of objects; brings objects to mouth; transfers objects from hand to hand	Rolls front to back; sits with support	Holds bottle when feeding; looks for removed objects (object permanence)	Turns in response to name; babbles
8–10 months	Pokes at objects with finger; progresses from ulnar to pincer grasp	Sits unsupported; starts to crawl; pulls to stand	Waves bye-bye; finger feeds	Babbles using two-syllables; shouts
12 months	Bangs bricks together; throws objects	Cruises between objects; walks	Claps hands; displays stranger awareness	Says 'Mama' and 'Dada'; understands simple sentences
15 months	Uses pincer grip for small objects	Walks stably	Points and pulls, drinks from a cup	Jabbers; repeats words; understands words for some objects

18 months	Scribbles (see Figure 5.6); turns two or three pages of a book at a time; builds a tower of two or three cubes	Carries toys while walking; runs unstably	Holds a cup in both hands; feeds self (see Figure 5.7)	Points to named body parts and common objects (e.g. 'door'); follows one-step requests
2 years	Turns pages of a book singly; copies a line	Runs stably	Plays alone (see Figure 5.8); eats with a fork and spoon	Says two-word sentences; has a 50-word vocabulary
2.5–3 years	Builds a tower of six to eight cubes; copies a circle	Climbs stairs one at a time; kicks a ball	Begins toilet training; puts on shoes and underwear	Says three- or four-word sentences; follows two-step requests
3.5–4 years	Builds a tower of nine or ten cubes; draws a person with arms and legs; copies a square	Pedals a tricycle; jumps well; hops	Eats with a knife and fork; toilets self unassisted	Asks lots of 'why' questions; counts to 10; uses the past tense
5 years	Copies a triangle; writes own name; does up buttons	Stands on one foot; comes down stairs one at a time	Chooses own friends; role plays	Counts to 20

Table 5.1 Developmental milestones.

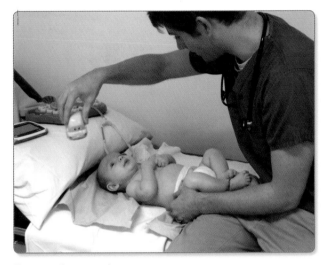

Figure 5.1 Fixes on an object.

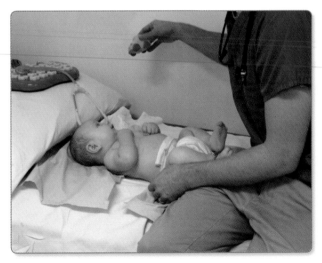

Figure 5.2 Follows an object through 45°.

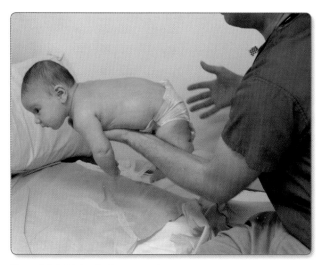

Figure 5.3 Holds head in line in ventral suspension.

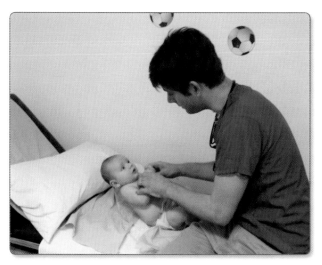

Figure 5.4 No head lag on pull to sit.

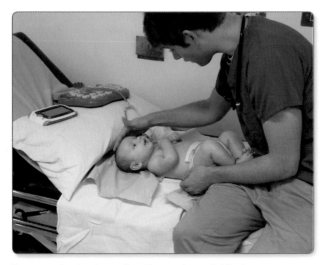

Figure 5.5 Social smiles at a face. (Also note how to feel for the anterior fontanelle in this photograph.)

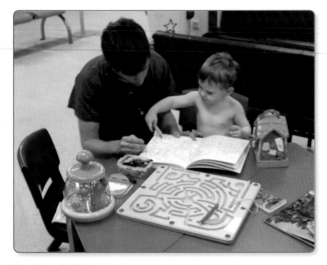

Figure 5.6 Scribbles.

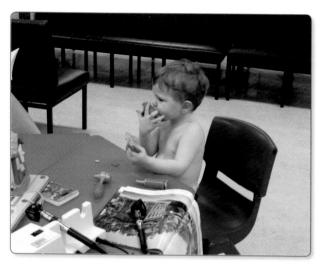

Figure 5.7 Feeds self.

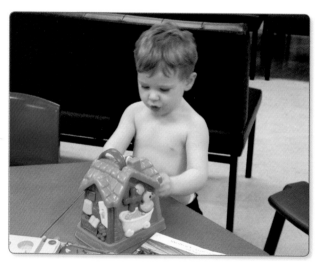

Figure 5.8 Plays alone.

The key to assessing development is to allow the child to demonstrate the skills that he or she can perform in turn, within one developmental domain, until a skill is reached that cannot be done – e.g. rolling, then sitting, crawling, standing, walking, running. A child unable to walk at 6 months is normal, whereas it would be considered abnormal at 18 months.

Assessing gross motor control at 1 year
Start by observing the child:
- simple observation may allow the entire examination to be performed – take a few seconds to watch what the child is doing
- if the child is sitting up playing with a toy, watch how the child is sitting – is the child leaning on their hands or sitting up unsupported?

Initially try to involve the parent in the assessment. For example, if the parent offers the child another toy just out of reach, how does the child get to it - by crawling, rolling, pulling to a standing position, cruising across the cot or walking across the cot? Or does the child sit and cry in frustration?

If this approach does not work, then approach the child. If the child is sitting in the cot it is reasonable to pull the child to stand and ascertain if he or she is stable holding the cot edges. If the child is stable, bring him or her out of the cot to the floor and see if the child will walk from you to the parent. If not, place the child on the front and see if he or she rolls on to the back and sits up (when tempted by a toy).

Clinical scenario

An assessment of gross motor skills in a 1-year-old boy shows that he can sit unsupported and will crawl towards a toy. He can also pull to stand, but he is unhappy when the toy is removed and will not cruise between objects. This represents a gross motor developmental age of approximately 10 months.

Assessing fine motor control at 3 years
The following steps should be performed:
1. begin by saying hello and ask the child his or her name – this enables you to assess hearing and speech.

2. offer the child a pencil and paper; start by watching how the child reaches out for the pencil – is there a mature radial pincer grip or an immature ulnar grasp?
3. now see what the child is able to draw – a 3-year-old would be expected to draw a line or to copy a circle but not to copy a square or a triangle

> ## Clinical scenario
>
> A 3-year-old girl has the facial appearance characteristic of Down syndrome (trisomy 21). When prompted, she says hello but doesn't say her name. When given a pencil and paper, she exhibits an immature grasp and begins scribbling on the paper. She is unable to copy a circle, leaves the table and runs unstably to her mother. This reflects fine motor development consistent with an 18-month-old child and is probably a delay secondary to trisomy 21.

5.3 Clinical scenarios

Developmental delay can present in a single domain, across multiple domains, or as global delay across all four domains. Global delay is almost invariably due to a central nervous system problem such as cerebral palsy (see Chapter 9).

> ## Clinical insight
>
> Hearing may be impaired in children with Down syndrome because they are susceptible to recurrent middle ear infections.

Brain	Cerebral palsy Neonatal stroke
Spinal cord	Spinal muscular atrophy
Neuromuscular junction	Myasthenia gravis
Muscle	Muscular dystrophy (Duchenne muscular dystrophy, Becker muscular dystrophy)
Global causes of weakness or hypotonia	Down syndrome (trisomy 21) Prader–Willi syndrome Hypothyroidism

Table 5.2 Differentials of gross motor delay in a 9-month old.

A 9-month-old girl who is not sitting

This is a gross motor problem. Motor skills require input from brain, spinal cord, motor neurone, neuromuscular junction and muscle (see Chapter 9). Therefore, the differential diagnosis is based on each of these structures.

Differential diagnosis

Possible causes of gross motor delay in a 9-month old to consider are given in **Table 5.2**.

Further information

The girl is the first child of non-consanguineous parents. She was born at 39 weeks' gestation following a normal pregnancy. Antenatal scans and blood tests (including screening for Down syndrome) were normal. She was breast-fed until 5 months.

Developmental assessment

Inspection   The differential diagnosis is quite broad but initial inspection will rule out some of the options. The child is lying flat on the examination couch, moving all four limbs normally and spontaneously. She is not dysmorphic. Therefore, cerebral palsy, stroke, Down syndrome and Prader–Willi syndrome can be ruled out.

The girl's facial expression is normal, although she looks a little wide-eyed – this rules out myasthenia gravis, in which the eyelids appear drooping. There is no maternal history of thyroid problems, and the newborn screening for hypothyroidism (on the Guthrie test card) was normal.

Examination   On examination, the child is markedly hypotonic. The most common forms of muscular dystrophy are X-linked disorders and are therefore unlikely in a female (see Chapter 15); moreover, hypotonia is not a feature of these disorders, and they rarely present in the first year of life.

Diagnosis   The girl has spinal muscular atrophy – an autosomal-recessive genetic disorder in which there is progressive death of motor neurones in the anterior horn of the spinal cord, resulting in progressive weakness. In this case the child presents with motor delay because she is not strong enough to sit.

Genetic testing confirms the diagnosis.

A 24-month-old boy who is not walking

A family come to the general paediatric clinic because their son is 24 months old and is still not walking.

Differential diagnosis

The boy has a delay in the gross motor domain. The differential diagnosis is the same as in the case above, with two additional possibilities:

- constitutional, or familial, delay
- severe rickets

Further information

The parents have noticed the boy cannot get up from the sitting position, but when they lift him up, he can stand steadily and cruise around furniture. He crawled initially and he now bottom-shuffles. He is an only child, and his mother carries him everywhere. It is of note that the father walked late (at 15 months). The child was not premature and has had no other illnesses

Developmental assessment

Inspection The boy is not dysmorphic. He scribbles with a colouring pencil and turns pages two at a time. He says two-word sentences.

Examination On examination, he can be seen to have very bulky calf muscles, and when he is put on the floor, he cannot stand up and has to be pulled to stand. He has an exaggerated lumbar lordosis. There are no features of rickets (such as swollen tender wrists or 'rickety rosary').

Diagnosis The creatinine kinase level is 8000 IU/L. Genetic testing confirms Duchenne muscular dystrophy. The mother is also tested and is not a carrier; it is a new mutation. A subsequent male child is unaffected.

A 30-month-old girl with speech delay

A family is referred to the paediatric clinic by the GP. The parents are concerned because their daughter is not saying words.

Differential diagnosis

Speech depends on environmental stimulation, normal hearing, the ability to process sounds, central generation of speech in the brain, and expression of speech using the muscles of the larynx and the mouth.

The main causes of speech delay are shown in **Table 5.3**.

Further information

The girl is the first child of parents with normal hearing. She was born at 34 weeks' gestation following a spontaneous onset of labour. There were no neonatal concerns noted, although she did receive antibiotic prophylaxis (gentamicin and penicillin) for 48 hours after birth. She did not require phototherapy for jaundice.

Her gross motor development and her fine motor development have been normal, and she walked at 11 months.

Developmental assessment

Inspection She does not appear dysmorphic. She makes babbling sounds and says 'Dada' and 'Baba'. She runs stably and will kick a ball. She is very interested in people and objects and watches people intently as they speak.

Hearing	Genetic deafness Congenital infection (cytomegalovirus, rubella) Ototoxic drugs (aminoglycosides)
Central processing	Cerebral palsy Kernicterus Autistic spectrum disorder
Generation of speech	Cleft palate Bulbar palsy

Table 5.3 Causes of speech delay.

Examination If handed a pencil she will scribble, and if asked to pick up a pencil and draw she will do so. If asked to collect a pencil that is hidden under the table she does not do so, and plays on her own instead. When her name is called from behind a screen she does not turn to look.

Diagnosis It is suspected that the reason for her speech delay is deafness. This diagnosis is confirmed on formal audiology testing. The maternal blood results at the time of the first antenatal are checked and show that her mother was not immune to cytomegalovirus (CMV). However, the Guthrie blood spot card shows that the girl was CMV-positive at birth.

The cause of the girl's deafness is congenital CMV infection. This may also be the cause of the premature birth, although other features of congenital CMV (e.g. low birth weight) were not noted. It is possible that the gentamicin (an aminoglycoside antibiotic) may also have contributed to the deafness.

> # Clinical insight
>
> Key points from this chapter:
> - keep a summary of the developmental milestones, or learn them – without this knowledge it is difficult to do a developmental assessment
> - practise developmental assessments – they are usually best done in a playroom, with siblings of patients if necessary

The respiratory system

The lungs have a limited repertoire of responses to disease – cough, breathlessness and wheeze. Respiratory problems in children often have an infectious cause; and in susceptible children infections can trigger wheezing. Wheezing may also be due to having inhaled a substance, such as pollen or traffic fumes, that other children can inhale without any problems. An important genetic cause of lung pathology – as well as a shortened lifespan – is cystic fibrosis, most commonly seen in Caucasian populations. The probable diagnoses of respiratory illness depend on the age of the child:

- babies are likely to have pneumonia or bronchiolitis
- toddlers may have inhaled a foreign body
- older children are likely to have asthma

6.1 Common presentations

The way in which a respiratory illness presents depends on which part of the respiratory tract that is affected. The key presentations in paediatrics are:

- stridor
- cough
- wheeze
- breathlessness

Stridor

Stridor is a noise made on inspiration that emanates from the larynx.

Differential diagnosis

The key differential diagnoses of stridor (**Table 6.1**) are:

- croup
- inhaled foreign body
- laryngomalacia
- epiglottitis

Viral infection – croup (laryngotracheobronchitis)
Inhaled foreign body – toys, food
Laryngomalacia – underdeveloped cartilage in the airway wall, which collapses during inspiration, thereby causing turbulent airflow (and therefore sound)
Bacterial infection – epiglottitis, caused by Haemophilus influenza type B; less common in countries that have introduced a Haemophilus vaccination programme

Table 6.1 Causes of stridor in children.

Croup

Pathology Croup is caused by a viral infection affecting the larynx and adjacent structures – croup is also called laryngotracheobronchitis. The airways become swollen and narrow, so that the normal, smooth and silent laminar airflow is disrupted and the airflow becomes turbulent and noisy.

Clinical features There is inspiratory stridor and (as a result of the swollen vocal cords) a harsh 'barking' cough. There may also be signs of respiratory distress (**Table 6.2**) if airflow is more limited. The illness usually lasts 24–36 hours, and corticosteroids may be required to decrease the swelling.

Inhaled foreign body

Pathology Small children often explore objects with their mouths, and they may inhale (aspirate) small objects, such as toys or pieces of food, which can become lodged in the airway.

Clinical features The inhalation may have been witnessed, but if not the clue in the history is a sudden onset of coughing, distress and stridor.

Treatment The foreign body must be removed, either immediately using an emergency forced manoeuvre (the Heimlich manoeuvre) or by laryngoscopy or bronchoscopy.

Increased respiratory rate
Nasal flare
Head bobbing
Tracheal tug
Chest recessions (subcostal, intercostal, supraclavicular)
Abdominal paradoxical movement
Tachycardia
Decreased level of consciousness
Pallor
Cyanosis
Hypotension

Table 6.2 Signs of respiratory distress.

Laryngomalacia

Pathology Laryngomalacia occurs when the cartilaginous walls of the upper airway are not sufficiently strong and collapse inwards on inspiration. This causes turbulent airflow and hence a soft inspiratory stridor.

Clinical features A soft inspiratory stridor may be constant or intermittent. The cartilaginous weakness is often anterior and the noise may be louder if the child is lying down or is upset and distressed or crying. When the child is asleep the muscle tone in the airway is decreased and there may be more stridor. As the child grows the airway increases in strength and the laryngomalacia resolves itself.

Diagnosis is usually clinical, but it can be made using fibreoptic laryngoscopy.

Epiglottitis

Pathology Epiglottitis is a bacterial infection of the epiglottis, caused by *Haemophilus influenzae*. It is much rarer than it used to be in countries that have introduced the *Haemophilus influenza* type B (Hib) vaccine.

Clinical features The child with epiglottitis looks very unwell, is flushed, and sits forwards holding the head forwards to maintain the airway patency. Swallowing is extremely painful and so the child drools saliva. There is stridor.

It is important not to examine the throat as this may cause the airway to occlude.

Cough

Cough is a very non-specific symptom and can occur as a result of any pathology at any site in the respiratory tract – cough is one of the clinical features of most respiratory pathologies. However, the timing of the cough and its associated features (such as the age of the patient and other symptoms) can give clues to the diagnosis. A few of the many possible causes of cough are considered in the following sections.

Differential diagnosis

Where cough is the prominent symptom, consider:

* asthma
* gastro-oesophageal reflux
* habitual cough

Asthma

Pathology The airway in asthma is hyper-responsive and reacts to antigens that are normally innocuous (e.g. pollen, dust, grass, pets) by contracting and narrowing. In the small airways this causes turbulent airflow, which is heard as wheeze. The inflammation in the airways can also trigger coughing.

Clinical features Asthma may be diagnosed around the age of 3 or 4 years. Children may wheeze before 4 years of age, but this is often in response to a viral infection (viral-induced wheeze). The first sign of asthma may be coughing at night, which can wake the child from sleep. There may also be wheezing (see below).

Treatment Treatment involves the use of bronchodilators (to relax the smooth muscle of the airways) and corticosteroids (to decrease inflammation).

Gastro-oesophageal reflux

Pathology Children have a short oesophagus and a weak lower oesophageal sphincter, and they drink large volumes of milk relative to their size, often lying flat after a large feed. Therefore stomach contents can easily reflux back into the oesophagus and the mouth. This may irritate the larynx and cause coughing.

Clinical features A child with gastro-oesophageal reflux has a persistent cough, which occurs mostly following feeds. There may also be a history of vomiting. Unlike the cough of asthma, which occurs predominantly at night, the cough of reflux occurs during daytime sleep as well.

Habitual cough

Pathology A habitual cough is a cough that arises out of habit, although it may have its origins in a preceding upper respiratory tract infection. There is no associated airway pathology.

Clinical features A habitual cough is commoner in older children and younger adolescents than in young children. It is a dry, non-productive cough, and it is not associated with any objective clinical signs such as wheeze or tachypnoea. It may be very persistent and attract a lot of concern from parents.

Treatment Once a diagnosis has been made, the treatment is to try to ignore it. Some children and families may require psychological support.

Wheeze

Wheeze is described as a 'musical' sound that emanates from the chest. It can sometimes be heard without the need for a stethoscope. Wheeze is caused by airflow in the lungs being disrupted by airway narrowing. This narrowing causes normal laminar airflow to become turbulent and to vibrate and cause noise. Wheeze is often worse on expiration because the airways normally narrow on breathing out.

Not everything that wheezes is asthma – but everything that wheezes is airway narrowing. For example, an inhaled foreign body will narrow the airways, resulting in wheeze. So will the inhalation of a noxious substance, as may occur when a teenager experiments with glue-sniffing. However, the commoner differentials are listed below.

Differential diagnoses

The list of differential diagnoses is based on the age of the child:

- bronchiolitis (in babies and children up to 1 year of age)
- virus-induced wheeze (in children aged between 1 and 3 or 4 years)
- asthma (in older children)

Bronchiolitis

Pathology Bronchiolitis is a viral lower respiratory tract infection occurring in babies and children up to 1 year of age. It begins with upper respiratory symptoms – a high-pitched cough and coryza (runny nose). As the infection spreads down the respiratory tract the bronchi and bronchioles become inflamed, oedematous and filled with mucus. The commonest pathogen is respiratory syncytial virus, although there are many others, including influenza A virus, influenza B virus, parainfluenza virus, adenovirus and the rhinoviruses.

Clinical features In addition to an initial cough and coryza, there may be pronounced sneezing. As the infection spreads to the chest there will be wheeze and shortness of breath, with periods of apnoea in more severe cases. Babies will have problems breathing while feeding, and they may vomit. The illness is usually worst between day 4 and day 6, and it lasts about 10 days in total, although the cough may persist for weeks afterwards. Auscultation reveals widespread crackles and wheezing that changes in nature from minute to minute as mucus moves around in the chest.

Viral-induced wheeze

Pathology Viral-induced wheeze is a viral lower respiratory tract infection that occurs in children between the ages of 1 year and 3 or 4 years. The causative organisms are the same as for bronchiolitis (see above); the difference is that the child is larger, resulting in different signs and symptoms, predominantly wheeze. As the viral infection spreads into the airways they become inflamed and narrowed, causing airflow limitation and wheezing.

Clinical features There will be cough and coryza, but the main features are wheezing together with signs of respiratory distress (see **Table 6.2**), which arise as the child generates a large negative intrathoracic pressure in an effort to get air through the narrow airways.

Treatment Treatment involves the use of bronchodilators (e.g. salbutamol, ipratropium, aminophylline) and anti-inflammatory agents (e.g. montelukast, corticosteroids).

Asthma

Pathology For a discussion of the pathology of asthma, see above. Asthma can be diagnosed after 3 or 4 years of age, once a child wheezes or has a persistent cough without a clear viral trigger.

Clinical features The clinical features are wheeze together with the signs of respiratory distress outlined in **Table 6.2**.
    Chronic asthma may result in a barrel-shaped chest (caused by chronic hyperinflation of the lungs) or a Harrison sulcus (an in-drawing of the skin at the lower costal margin).

Breathlessness

Breathlessness is a lay term that encapsulates difficulty in breathing (dyspnoea) with rapid breathing (tachypnoea). It is a sensation driven by the brainstem sensing raised carbon dioxide levels in the blood (hypercapnia). In chronic respiratory illness this reflex may diminish, in which case the drive to breathe comes from the partial pressure of oxygen in the bloodstream.

The excretion of carbon dioxide depends on alveolar ventilation, so anything that prevents air reaching the alveoli may cause breathlessness.

Differential diagnosis

The differential diagnosis of breathlessness includes:

- viral-induced wheeze and asthma
- pneumonia
- pleural effusion or empyema

Viral-induced wheeze and asthma

Pathology and management For a discussion of the pathology, see above. It is important to realise that viral wheeze and asthma can cause profound limitation to airflow, and in severe cases positive pressure ventilation may be required to achieve adequate alveolar gas exchange.

Pneumonia

Pathology Pneumonia is an infection of the lung parenchyma – whereas viral wheeze affects the conducting airways, in pneumonia there is infection in the alveolar spaces. It is usually viral or bacterial in aetiology.

Clinical features and management Pneumonia causes fever and tachypnoea, and there may be dyspnoea. There may also be associated systemic symptoms of infection, such as vomiting, loss of appetite and tachycardia.

Auscultation may reveal crackles (crepitations), which are caused by air bubbling through fluid or pus within the lung. On chest X-ray, patches of consolidation or segmental collapse may be visible.

Supportive therapy (oxygen and fluids) and antibiotics should be given.

Pleural effusion or empyema

Pathology   A pleural effusion is a collection of fluid in the pleural space – between the lung and the chest wall. An empyema is a pleural effusion that consists of pus. In children, pleural effusion and empyema occur secondary to infection. (In adults they can be associated with malignancy, but this is rarely the case in children.)

Clinical features and management   There may be shortness of breath and pain on inspiration. Because it can be painful, children with an effusion or an empyema often sit with the spine curved to the side of the effusion.

On examination there is decreased air entry (because the sound of air entering the lung cannot pass through fluid), and there is a 'stony-dull' percussion note.

The patient will have a high fever and appear unwell. Antibiotics should be given, and if the effusion is large enough, drainage will be needed.

6.2 Respiratory examination

Wash your hands and introduce yourself.

General inspection

The examination in children starts during the history, and most of the respiratory assessment can be done from a distance, while the infant or child is sitting with the parent and not being distracted by other adults.

Exposure

Formal inspection should be done with the child appropriately exposed and positioned. This depends on the child's age and mood.

A baby is ideally examined lying on the back on an open nappy.

It is usually best to have a toddler on a parent's lap. The undressing of a toddler is best left to the parents, and if this appears to be causing the child to become upset, inspection should first be carried out with the child still clothed.

An older child or adolescent is examined as an adult would be, sitting up on a couch at an angle of 45–60° and undressed to the waist (with consideration for modesty in young adults).

Is the child well or unwell?

Observe for signs of respiratory distress (see **Table 6.2**). Measure the respiratory rate from the end of the bed (count the number of breaths over 30 seconds and double it).

Consider how the child looks – is the child sitting up happily on the bed or on a parent's lap? Or is the child lying on the bed, mostly hidden behind an oxygen mask, drawing deep breaths and looking tired?

Oxygen is important for the brain, so an impaired level of consciousness may imply hypoxia. Hypoxic children may be combative or irritable. Check how high the oxygen flow rate is set, and that the mask fits appropriately.

Around the bed

Look around the bed for clues. Is there a saturation monitor on, and what does it show? Are there inhalers, spacers, peak-flow meters or tissues around the bed? Has a parent brought in the child's home oxygen cylinder or a home nebuliser?

The hands

Look at the hands for the following signs:

- clubbing
- cyanosis
- pulse
- asterixis

Clubbing

Clubbing is a swelling at the base of the nailbed.

Approach Ask the child to hold out the hands and inspect the nailbed.

Appearance If there is clubbing, the nail bed may be swollen, and the angle formed by the junction of the nail bed with the skin, which is usually concave, is convex.

Associated conditions In respiratory paediatrics, clubbing is associated with chronic hypoxia – the two common causes are
- cystic fibrosis
- chronic lung disease of prematurity

Cyanosis

Cyanosis is a blue discoloration to the skin caused by an increased amount of deoxygenated blood in the capillaries.

Cyanosis reveals itself when >5g/dL of blood is not carrying oxygen. Therefore, a child with anaemia may be hypoxic but will not appear cyanosed because there is not enough deoxygenated haemoglobin in the circulation. This is particularly pertinent in ex-premature babies, who often have low haemoglobin levels (the anaemia of prematurity).

Appearance The fingernails may appear blue or grey. Look at the fingernails and compare their colour to your own to recognise subtle peripheral cyanosis (**Figure 6.1**).

Associated conditions Cyanosis is associated with inadequate oxygenation of the blood, and therefore any cause of acute or chronic hypoxia will cause cyanosis (e.g. severe acute asthma, pulmonary hypertension, cystic fibrosis, complex congenital heart disease).

Pulse

A peripheral assessment of the heart rate and stroke volume should be made.

Approach In a baby, feel for the pulse at the brachial artery (medially in the antecubital fossa). In an older child take the radial pulse as in an adult. Feel for 30 seconds and double the rate to reach a value for beats per minute

Is there a tachycardia or bradycardia? Compare to normal values for age (see Chapter 2). The pulse may have a small

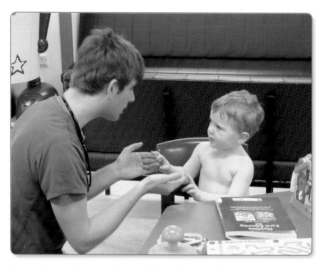

Figure 6.1 Looking at the fingernails for clubbing and for cyanosis.

volume if there has been fluid loss, or it may be 'bounding' in sepsis.

Associated conditions Respiratory compromise may be associated with a tachycardia; if the compromise is severe and the child is decompensating, there may be a bradycardia. If there appears to be respiratory compromise, the blood pressure should be measured.

Asterixis

Asterixis is a rhythmic flapping movement at the wrists.

Approach Ask the child to hold the arms out straight in front and to hold the palms out, facing forward, with the wrists cocked backwards. If asterixis is present, the hands will 'beat' forwards.

Associated conditions Asterixis is associated with acidosis, either as a result of a metabolic problem (e.g. liver failure) or as a result of respiratory pathology causing carbon dioxide retention.

The face and neck

The face and neck can give valuable clues during the respiratory examination. Look at:

- the eyes
- the mouth and tongue
- the lymph nodes

Approach and associations Gently look inside the lower eyelids to assess the colour. They are pale in anaemia. Ask the child to stick out the tongue (**Figure 6.2**) to check for cyanosis (a blue coloration to the skin); it can be useful to compare the colour to that of your thumbnail.

Palpate for lymph nodes, which are often the hallmark of upper airway infections such as tonsillitis. Palpate all of the lymph node areas, including behind the clavicles and in the armpits (see Chapter 10). Assess whether the nodes are

- tender or painless

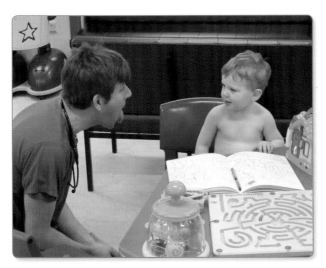

Figure 6.2 Younger children might need some prompting to stick their tongue out.

- fixed or mobile
- limited to one site or distributed in multiple areas

The chest

Chest examination follows the sequence:
- inspection
- palpation
- percussion
- auscultation

Inspection

Respiratory distress Inspect for signs of respiratory distress (**Figure 6.3**; see also **Table 6.2**).

Chest shape Look for abnormalities of the chest shape:
- pectus excavatum
- pectus carinatum

Assess the anterior–posterior diameter of the chest; this may be increased in chronic respiratory disease.

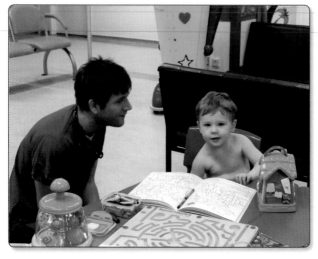

Figure 6.3 Taking the opportunity to do a general inspection of the chest.

Chest wall abnormalities Check for a Harrison sulcus – a subcostal area of indrawn skin with flaring of the ribs at the costal margin. It develops as the result of chronic increased work of breathing, and is a sign of poorly managed asthma.

Palpation

Chest expansion It is important to assess chest expansion if hyperexpansion is suspected, but to do so requires a co-operative patient:

- the examiner places his or her hands on the front of the child's chest with the fingers pointing upwards
- the child is asked to inhale fully and then to exhale; a full expiration should be encouraged
- the examiner then brings the thumbs together and asks the child to take a full inspiration again; the thumbs should end up a good distance apart

The actual distance depends on the size of the patient, and (unlike in adults), there is not a 'one-size-fits-all' rule for the number of centimetres that should separate the thumbs by the end of the test. If the thumbs have barely moved then this is obviously abnormal.

Repeat the test on the patient's back (which may be easier anyway with teenage girls) by leaning past the patient and placing the palm of the hand on the back, with the fingers pointing downwards.

Apex beat Palpate to assess the position of the apex of the heart, which may not be in the left side of the chest (e.g. in dextrocardia or situs invertus).

Lymphadenopathy Palpate for lymphadenopathy (see Chapter 10), including in the axillae (**Figure 6.4**)

Percussion

Percuss over each lung lobe (**Figure 6.5**) for:

- areas of dullness (indicating fluid or solid lung – consolidation)
- hyper-resonance (indicating air in the pleural space).

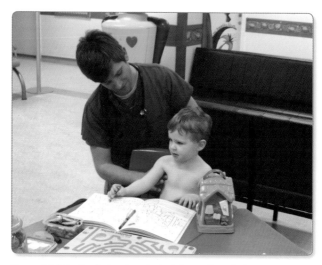

Figure 6.4 Palpating for lymph nodes (including in the axillae).

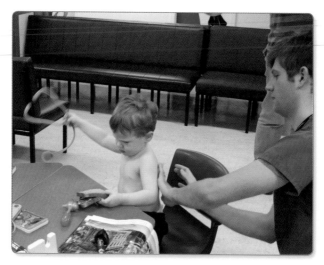

Figure 6.5 Percussing for areas of dullness or hyper-resonance.

It is important to assess mid-zone pathology by percussing in the axillae.

Auscultation

Listen to the chest, comparing one side with the other on the front and back, and crucially in the axillae (otherwise mid-zone pathology may be missed) (**Figure 6.6**). Auscultatory sounds in children are multiple, multilayered and often confusing.

Crackles Crackles are caused by air bubbling through something – either pus (in infection) or water (in oedema).
Airway oedema occurs secondary either to:
- decreased oncotic pressure in the blood and transmural osmosis (such as occurs in cardiac failure or nephrotic syndrome)
- inflammation (such as occurs in asthma or viral infections).

Wheeze Wheeze is caused by turbulent airflow in small airways.

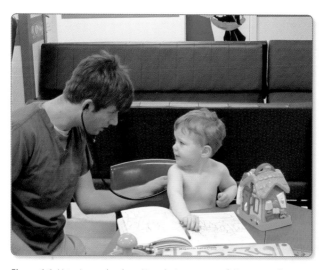

Figure 6.6 Listening to the chest. Note the importance of distraction when getting a child comfortable for a physical examination.

Bronchial breathing Bronchial breathing is the sound made when there are consolidated alveoli next to a patent small airway. On auscultation the sound of air rushing in and out of the airway is heard, but not the gentler (though louder) noise of the alveoli expanding. The sound is described as sounding high and harsh. There are audio files of bronchial breathing available on the internet.

No air entry No air entry occurs in the following situations:
- collapsed lung
- fluid between the lung and the stethoscope (i.e. an effusion)
- consolidation (i.e. airways full of pus, so that no air can move)
- pneumothorax

These four entities may be differentiated using percussion and tactile and vocal fremitus. If the lung is consolidated, vocal resonance is increased; if there is a pleural effusion, it is decreased.

Interpreting multiple signs

It is rare to hear sounds of one, single pathology in a set of lungs. A typical patient might be a coryzal 3-year-old child, wheezing and short of breath as a result of an upper respiratory tract infection and a viral-induced wheeze. Possible signs found on auscultation and their likely meaning are given in **Table 6.3**.

Examination findings should be considered in the context of the history: 'Put an ear to the patient having already thought about what might be heard.'

Further examination and bedside tests

Further examination

Palpate the abdomen; the liver may be displaced downwards by hyperexpanded lungs. It is usual to feel a 1 cm liver edge in babies and infants. It is appropriate to carry on and perform an ENT examination (see Chapter 13).

Finish by offering to weigh and measure the height of the child. Plot the values on the appropriate centile charts.

Sign on auscultation	Interpretation
Thumping heart rate	Indicates that the child is ill
Snuffly noise that sounds a bit like snoring	Snuffly snoring noises originate from the upper airways. This can be demonstrated by holding the stethoscope up in front of the child's mouth and listening to noisy mouth breathing and nasal bubblings as they happen in expiration. All the noises heard in the chest are transmitted inwards on inspiration.
Scattered wheeze (i.e. heard throughout the chest) that comes and goes, often between individual breaths	Wheeze represents narrowed airways
Fine crackles	Indicates the presence of fluid in the airways, with bubbles being formed as air goes in
Bronchial noises	Heard if the stethoscope is placed over a main bronchus when trying to hear heart sounds – a normal finding in such a situation. Bronchial noises are abnormal if heard in the periphery of the lungs and imply consolidation

Table 6.3 Interpreting multiple respiratory signs: auscultation signs and their meaning in a coryzal 3-year-old child who is wheezing and short of breath with a viral upper respiratory tract infection.

Relevant investigations

Simple bedside tests done as part of a respiratory examination are:
- saturation monitoring
- peak flow monitoring

You should ask for these tests and be able to interpret the results in the appropriate setting. In particular, you should always ask for them if there any concerns about wheeze – compare the results to the charts showing 'best predicted value for height'.

Learn how to show a child how to use a peak flow meter by observing their use in clinic or on the wards.

6.3 Clinical scenarios

A 7-year-old boy who is coughing at night

A 7-year-old boy is referred to the paediatric outpatients department by his GP. The school nurse has telephoned, because he keeps falling asleep in class. His mother is concerned because he is 'coughing all night'. The boy and his mother have recently moved in with her new partner, who is a smoker. The boy has mild hay fever, and he had eczema as a baby, although he has grown out of it.

Differential diagnosis

Children may fall asleep in class because they are not sleeping properly at night. Consider:

- poor sleep hygiene, perhaps caused by a lack of routine at bedtime or by having a television or a computer in the bedroom
- obstructed breathing and sleep apnoea with repeated waking, which may be due to chronic tonsillitis
- coughing at night, which may be due to asthma, rhinitis or allergy
- gastro-oesophageal reflux, which may irritate the throat and cause coughing

Further information

On further questioning, you learn that his bedtimes have been disrupted by moving house, although only occasionally. He does not snore. He is a little too old to develop reflux and he has not had problems with it in the past, so a pH probe does not seem a reasonable investigation. Because he has hay fever and has had eczema and is now being exposed to cigarette smoke, you suspect asthma. This diagnosis is confirmed on examination when you hear an occasional patchy wheeze.

Concluding diagnosis

This boy has asthma. You recommend smoking cessation advice for his mother's new partner and prescribe a salbutamol inhaler for use for before bedtime.

A 3-month-old boy with poor feeding

A 3-month-old boy is brought in by ambulance from a nearby GP surgery. He has been unwell with a snuffly nose for 2 days, and today he has been able to breast-feed for only 5 minutes at a time because he gets out of breath. His mother thinks that he may have stopped breathing at one point for about 10 seconds.

On examination the airway is patent, oxygen saturation is 92%, breathing is rapid with chest recessions, and auscultation demonstrates bilateral soft crackles with patchy wheezing. The liver is displaced 2 cm inferiorly. Cardiovascular status is normal.

Diagnosis

The challenge here is not the diagnosis – this is the classical presentation of acute bronchiolitis, a viral lower respiratory tract infection that affects babies under 1 year. It is often caused by respiratory syncytial virus.

The important decision here surrounds management; is it safe to send this child home? Babies with bronchiolitis can be safely managed at home as long as they are feeding sufficiently and have adequate respirations (as shown by acceptable oxygen saturations and only mild respiratory distress). The role of hospital admission is to provide supportive care (feeding or oxygen) if the baby requires it. In this boy, the oxygen saturations are quite low (92%) and there is a history of what may be apnoeas (pauses in breathing).

> ## Clinical insight
>
> Key points from this chapter:
> - respiratory illness is extremely common in children
> - the commonest aetiology is infection
> - know the signs of respiratory distress
> - consider the possible diagnoses before examining the child

Management plan
In view of these considerations, the baby is admitted for oxygen by nasal prongs and for feeding via a nasogastric tube.

The cardiovascular system

Cardiac disease presents in a wide variety of ways, including postnatal collapse, cyanosis, heart failure, syncope or, rarely, sudden death. Many cardiac lesions have an associated murmur, which can give a clue to the cause. A murmur may be an innocent finding (see clinical scenarios).

Most cardiac disease in childhood is congenital. Approximately eight per 1000 live births are affected, the commonest disorder being a ventricular septal defect (VSD), accounting for 30% of cases. Some children have very complex disease with multiple structural abnormalities being present together, which is beyond the scope of this book. Antenatal fetal scanning detects a significant number of these anomalies.

7.1 Common presentations

Common cardiovascular presentations include:
- cyanosis
- heart failure
- syncope or sudden death

Cyanosis

There are three main conditions in which the child may present with cyanosis:
- transposition of the great arteries (TGA)
- tetralogy of Fallot (ToF)
- atrioventricular septal defect (AVSD)

Transposition of the great arteries

Pathology In TGA, the venous and arterial systems are completely separate, for the aorta arises from the right ventricle and the pulmonary trunk arises from the left (**Figure 7.1**). An atrial septal defect (ASD) may also be present; this can allow some oxygenated blood to enter the systemic circulation. Without an ASD, the only way in which oxygenated blood can enter the systemic circulation is via the ductus arteriosus. In fetal life, this structure allows oxygenated blood to bypass the lungs and enter the systemic circulation (**Figure 7.2**), but it closes in the first week after birth.

Clinical features The infant with TGA always appears blue. In addition, if there is no ASD present, then once the ductus has closed the child is unable to get enough blood to the lungs, and so develops:

- low oxygen saturations
- tachycardia
- shock
- a raised plasma lactate level (as a result of anaerobic respiration)
- a murmur

Treatment Prostaglandin E is given urgently to keep the ductus arteriosus open temporarily while urgent surgical correction can be arranged. Corrective surgery is needed to 'switch' the great vessels.

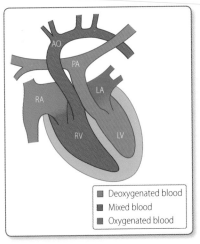

Figure 7.1 Transposition of the great arteries (TGA). Ao, aorta; LA, left atrium; LV, left ventricle; PA, pulmonary artery; RA, right atrium; RV, right ventricle.

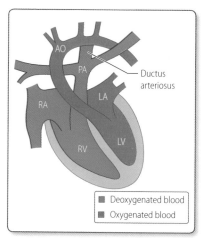

Figure 7.2 The ductus arteriosus. Ao, aorta; LA, left atrium; LV, left ventricle; PA, pulmonary artery; RA, right atrium; RV, right ventricle.

Deoxygenated blood
Oxygenated blood

Tetralogy of Fallot

Pathology The four features of the tetralogy (**Figure 7.3**) are:
- subpulmonary outflow tract obstruction
- over-riding aorta
- VSD
- right ventricular hypertrophy

In ToF, deoxygenated blood can enter the right ventricle as normal, but from here on there is a problem with blood flow. There is an obstruction to blood flow out of the right ventricle across the pulmonary valve. Some of this deoxygenated blood therefore flows via the path of least resistance, either across the VSD or out into the over-riding aorta and into the systemic arterial supply. The only way the blood can get back into the lungs is through the ductus arteriosus to the pulmonary artery, if the ductus is still open.

Clinical features Children with ToF are cyanosed, because the oxygenated blood is mixed with deoxygenated blood. They can suffer intermittent cyanotic spells, during which the pulmonary pressure increases temporarily, sending all the blood via the VSD and the over-riding aorta.

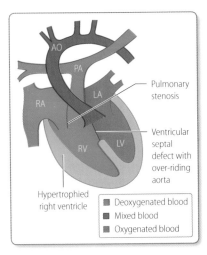

Figure 7.3 Tetralogy of Fallot (ToF). Ao, aorta; LA, left atrium; LV, left ventricle; PA, pulmonary artery; RA, right atrium; RV, right ventricle.

Pulmonary stenosis

Ventricular septal defect with over-riding aorta

Hypertrophied right ventricle

■ Deoxygenated blood
■ Mixed blood
■ Oxygenated blood

An infant who is born with severe ToF in which little or no blood can get across the pulmonary outflow obstruction is dependent on the ductus arteriosus. As with TGA (see above), once the ductus closes, the baby will collapse. Therefore, as with TGA, prostaglandin therapy is needed to keep the ductus open until urgent surgical correction can be performed.

Clinical insight

Any newborn infant who becomes cyanosed or shocked must be assessed immediately for the presence of a duct-dependent cardiac defect.

Atrioventricular septal defect

Pathology In AVSD, there is an abnormality in both the atrial septum and the ventricular septum. AVSD may occur as part of a multisystem disorder – AVSDs are associated with Down syndrome (trisomy 21), for example. Oxygenated and deoxygenated blood mix in the atria and again in the ventricles.

Clinical features AVSD presents in the neonatal period with a combination of cyanosis and heart failure. An ejection systolic murmur may be heard over the pulmonary region.

Heart failure

Heart failure is the term given to the group of symptoms that arise when there is inadequate supply of oxygen and nutrients to the tissues. Most cases of heart failure in children are due to an underlying congenital heart defect (see below), but there are also rarer acquired causes, such as acute viral myocarditis, in which a virus damages the myocardium.

In the commonest forms of congenital heart diseases [VSD, ASD and patent ductus arteriosus (PDA)], a left-to-right shunt of blood across the defect occurs. This can result in pulmonary overflow and wet lungs as well as decreased systemic output and inadequate perfusion of the systemic circulation. Almost all types of congenital heart disease can cause heart failure, including ToF as described above, but only the common causes are described below.

The key signs of heart failure in a baby are shown in **Table 7.1**. Common causes of heart failure are:

- ASD
- VSD
- PDA
- Coarctation of the aorta

> ### Clinical insight
>
> A baby who is having feeding difficulty with breathlessness must be assessed for heart failure as well as respiratory illness.

Early	Late
Poor feeding	Failure to thrive
Poor weight gain	Generalised oedema
Tachypnoea, especially during feeds	Ascites
Sweating during feeds	
A murmur	
Fine crackles on auscultation of the chest	
Hepatomegaly	

Table 7.1 Symptoms and signs in heart failure.

Atrial septal defect

Pathology In ASD there is a defect between the atria that allows blood to cross from the high-pressure (left) side to the low-pressure (right) side.

Clinical features Most commonly the diagnosis is suspected after an incidental finding of a murmur on clinical examination. The murmur is usually a pulmonary flow murmur caused by the increased volume of blood passing across the pulmonary valve as a result of the left-to-right shunt.

In addition, the pulmonary valve is held open for longer than normal, which results in a fixed splitting of the second heart sound (S2). Heart failure may also occur, with the features as listed above.

Ventricular septal defect

Pathology In VSD, there is a defect between the ventricles (**Figure 7.4**) that allows blood to cross from the high-pressure (left) side to the low-pressure (right) side. This may result in not

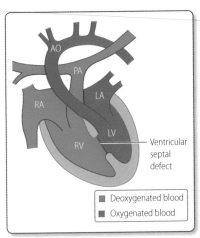

Figure 7.4 Ventricular septal defect (VSD). Ao, aorta; LA, left atrium; LV, left ventricle; PA, pulmonary artery; RA, right atrium; RV, right ventricle.

enough blood entering the systemic circulation (causing heart failure) and too much blood entering the pulmonary circulation (causing pulmonary oedema, resulting in tachypnoea).

Clinical features The infant with VSD classically presents with heart failure at around 6 weeks of age. This delayed presentation occurs because the right-sided pressures remain high for several weeks after the transition from fetal circulation and there is therefore little left-to-right flow of blood. Therefore, the classic murmur is often not present initially. However, once the right-sided pressures fall, there is significant left-to-right shunting of blood. In small VSDs, heart failure may not occur and in such cases the only clinical evidence of the defect is the murmur.

Over time, if the VSD is uncorrected, an increase in pulmonary pressure can occur, resulting in pulmonary hypertension. This reverses the flow of blood across the VSD so that there is right-to-left flow, causing deoxygenated blood to enter the systemic circulation, with resultant cyanosis. This is the Eisenmenger syndrome.

Patent ductus arteriosus

Pathology If the ductus arteriosus (see **Figure 7.2**) remains open (patent) instead as closing as it should do in the first few days of life, blood can flow from the high-pressure aorta into the low-pressure pulmonary circulation. PDA is commoner in infants born prematurely than in other infants.

Clinical features In PDA, there is a murmur, and babies may suffer from periodic oxygen desaturation and apnoea. The duct can be encouraged to close using medications (e.g. ibuprofen, indometacin), but surgical ligation may be required.

Coarctation of the aorta

Pathology Coarctation of the aorta (**Figure 7.5**) is caused by narrowing of the aorta at the site where the ductus arteriosus inserts into it.

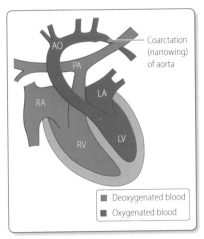

Figure 7.5 Coarctation of the aorta. Ao, aorta; LA, left atrium; LV, left ventricle; PA, pulmonary artery; RA, right atrium; RV, right ventricle.

Clinical features In neonates, coarctation of the aorta may present as collapse or heart failure. Older children may present with hypertension. Coarctation is sometimes diagnosed following an incidental detection of a murmur. In a neonate it can be a life-threatening condition if it causes collapse once the ductus arteriosus starts to close. Such an infant presents with shock, and immediate administration of prostaglandin is required to maintain patency of the ductus until urgent surgery can be performed.

If collapse does not occur on closure of the ductus, coarctation may remain asymptomatic and may be diagnosed only through the incidental detection of a murmur or when hypertension is discovered.

The murmur is an ejection systolic murmur, which can be heard all over the praecordium and may radiate to the carotids.

The cardinal clinical sign of coarctation is weak femoral pulses, with lower blood pressures in the legs than in the arms.

Syncope or sudden death

Cardiac disease may present itself as either syncope or sudden death at any age. Syncope, or 'fainting', occurs when there is a sudden fall in the cerebral perfusion pressure.

Sudden death is fortunately rare but is one of the main reasons for otherwise fit and seemingly healthy children to die suddenly, particularly during sporting activity.

The main causes are:

- arrhythmias
- cardiomyopathies

Arrhythmias

An arrhythmia is an abnormal cardiac rhythm. There are many types of arrhythmia; two that are important in general paediatric practice are:

- supraventricular tachycardia (SVT)
- long QT syndrome

Supraventricular tachycardia

Pathology   In SVT, there is an abnormal rhythm in the atria. This abnormal rhythm may originate in the sinus node or at another site. The atria beat rapidly and, if this rapid impulse is transmitted to the ventricle (either through the atrioventricular node or via another route), then the ventricles also beat rapidly – at above 180 beats per minute. Cardiac output may be decreased because the heart does not have time to fill and the stroke volume falls, and the blood supply to the brain suddenly decreases.

Clinical features   The patient may have an awareness of palpitations, or there may be a prodrome of nausea, changing vision or hearing loss preceding a faint. ECG shows a narrow complex tachycardia.

Long QT syndrome

Pathology   Long QT syndrome comprises a group of genetic disorders that affect surface membrane ion channels on the cardiac muscle. Children and adults with long QT syndrome can suffer from arrhythmias or asystole leading to sudden death.

Clinical features   In long QT syndrome, there may be a personal history of fainting and a family history of sudden unexplained death in young people, especially during exertion (such as swimming). The ECG shows a prolonged corrected QT interval (QTc). It is important to check the QTc on an ECG because family members can be screened if a disorder is identified.

Cardiomyopathy

Cardiomyopathy may be genetic or it may be an acute transient problem. Common causes include:

- inherited disease, e.g. hypertrophic obstructive cardiomyopathy (HOCM)
- acute viral cardiomyopathy
- acute vitamin D-deficiency cardiomyopathy

Pathology   In cardiomyopathy, the cardiac muscle is weakened, leading to a decrease in the amount of blood that the heart is able to pump. Heart failure may occur as a result.

HOCM is a familial disorder in which the myocardium is bulky and obstructs blood flow out of the heart.

Viruses such as Coxsackie A virus can directly infect the myocardium, causing it to become inflamed and decrease the power of the muscle contraction.

In severe rickets (caused by deficiency of vitamin D), heart failure may occur as a result of low serum calcium causing weak muscle contraction.

Clinical insight

Key points in the patient's history to look at when considering cardiac pathology in a child include:

- antenatal scans
- prematurity (e.g. PDA is commoner in premature infants)
- syndromes (e.g. AVSD may occur in Down syndrome)
- family history, affected parents or siblings
- consanguinous parents
- baby check
- feeding
- weight gain
- blue spells (a hallmark of ToF)

Clinical features

Cardiomyopathy usually presents with an enlarged heart and other signs of heart failure (**Table 7.1**). Inflamed heart muscle (as occurs in viral myocarditis, for example) also increases the risk of arrhythmias.

7.2 Cardiac examination

General inspection

Exposure

Examine a baby on a couch, an infant or toddler on the mother's lap, and an older child or adolescent as an adult, with the patient sitting up on a couch at 45°. Babies should be undressed to the nappy, and children and adolescents should be undressed to the waist (with appropriate sensitivity towards modesty in adolescents).

Around the bed

Look around the bed for any clues, such as saturation monitoring devices or infusions.

General assessment

Look at the child. Is the child dysmorphic? Is the child thin and malnourished? Check and plot the height or length, the weight and the head (occiptofrontal) circumference.

Is the child blue? Check the oxygen saturations.

Assess the respiratory rate and effort, and look for chest recessions (see Chapter 6). Look for any obvious scars.

Hands

The hands should be examined for:
- clubbing
- splinter haemorrhages
- pulses and blood pressure

Clubbing

Appearance   Clubbing is a swelling at the base of the nail bed.

Associated conditions Clubbing may be present in cyanotic congenital heart disease.

Splinter haemorrhages

Pathology Splinter haemorrhages are caused by small colonies of bacteria detaching from a colony on a cardiac valve in patients with valvular endocarditis and depositing in small capillary beds (such as in the fingers).

Appearance Splinter haemorrhages are small linear haemorrhages underneath the nail

Associated conditions Splinter haemorrhages may be visible in bacterial endocarditis (a bacterial infection on a heart valve or on the lining of the endocardium).

Small deposits of bacteria in the kidneys may cause microscopic haematuria; it is important to test the urine for blood if there is concern about bacterial endocarditis.

Pulses and blood pressure

In a baby or toddler, feel the pulse at the brachial artery (**Figure 7.6**). In an older child, a check of the radial pulse should suffice. Examine the pulse for rate, rhythm and volume, and for brachial–brachial or brachial–femoral delay in coarctation. Also assess the blood pressure at this point.

> **Clinical insight**
>
> It is vital to assess the femoral pulses when doing a cardiac examination on a baby.

Head and neck

Eyes

Check the conjunctivae for anaemia (they may be pale) and the sclerae for jaundice (icterus). Jaundice may be the result of haemolysis caused by a prosthetic heart valve.

Jugular venous pulse

If the child is able to sit up at 45° degrees, the jugular venous pressure (JVP) should be examined. In a baby, an enlarged liver is the 'examination equivalent' of a raised JVP. A raised

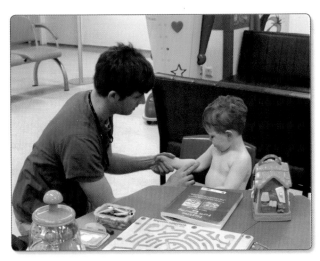

Figure 7.6 Feeling for the brachial pulse.

JVP suggests that the patient has raised right-sided heart pressures.

Mouth and tongue

Look at the underside of the tongue to assess for central cyanosis – a blue discoloration. Inspect the teeth – poor dentition may be an entry route for bacteria, resulting in infective endocarditis.

Praecordium

Stand back and inspect the patient again. In an examination setting, the chest inspection should give a wealth of information about what may subsequently be found on auscultation. Assess for a visible apex beat.

Look for any scars:

- a median sternotomy scar suggests that open heart surgery has been performed, e.g. VSD repair, arterial switch operation for TGA
- a left lateral thoracotomy scar (high and posterior in the axilla) suggests that a PDA ligation or Blalock-Taussig (BT) shunt has been performed

Palpate for the apex beat. If no apex beat can be felt on the left side, feel on the right side in case the patient has dextrocardia. Palpate for heaves and thrills; a right ventricular heave will be felt at the left sternal border. Thrills should be palpated for over the corresponding auscultatory valve areas (see below).

Auscultation

Auscultation is performed to assess heart sounds and to listen for murmurs.

Heart sounds

Apex Begin by listening at the apex (the mitral area) (**Figure 7.7**) to the cycle of heart sounds – 'ba-dum, ba-dum, ba-dum'. The rate is faster than in an adult, and the left main bronchus lies close by, so harsh breathing noises interfere with the heart sounds.

Tricuspid area Next, listen at the lower left sternal edge (the tricuspid area – approximately the fifth intercostal space), then

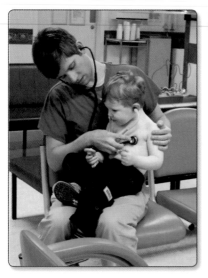

Figure 7.7 Listening at the apex.

at the upper left sternal edge (the pulmonary area – the second intercostal space), and finally at the upper right sternal border (the aortic area – the second intercostal space) (**Figure 7.8**).

Splitting of the second heart sound Listen for splitting of S2. S2 is made up of the aortic component (A2) and the pulmonary component (P2). The timing of these two components depends on inspiration and expiration. On inspiration, more blood enters the right ventricle (as systemic venous return is increased by the negative intrathoracic pressure). This results in greater filling in the right ventricle, and more blood is expelled across the pulmonary valve. Therefore, the pulmonary valve closes later – and P2 occurs after A2. The reverse occurs in expiration.

If the atrial pressures are abnormally high then ventricular filling is affected, and the splitting no longer varies with respiration, and S2 becomes 'fixed'. This fixed splitting of S2 occurs in an ASD when the right atrial pressure is increased because blood is flowing from the left atrium across the defect into the right atrium.

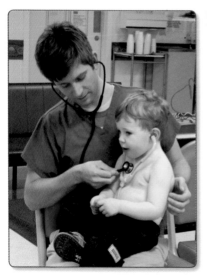

Figure 7.8 Listening at the aortic area.

Murmurs

Listen for any extra, abnormal sounds – murmurs. The cause of a murmur can be ascertained by listening for where it radiates to (**Table 7.2**).

Any murmur should be graded (**Table 7.3**).

Finishing the examination

Sit the patient forward and listen to the lung bases (**Figure 7.9**) for fine crackles (which may be heard in pulmonary oedema), and assess whether any murmurs radiate to the back. Press over the sacrum to assess for sacral oedema; in a patient who has been in bed for a prolonged period, oedema may have become redistributed to the sacral area.

Site of loudest volume	Timing	Radiation	Pathology
Apex	Pansystolic	To the axilla	VSD
Lower left sternal edge	Early systolic	Doesn't radiate	Innocent murmur
Pulmonary area	Pansystolic Ejection systolic	To the back	PDA; AVSD
Aortic area	Ejection systolic	To the carotid arteries; to the back	Coarctation of the aorta

Table 7.2 Heart murmurs by location. AVSD, atrioventricular septal defect; PDA, patent ductus arteriosus; VSD, ventricular septal defect.

Grade 1	Can be heard by an expert in a quiet room
Grade 2	Sounds quiet to a non-expert in a quiet room
Grade 3	Heard easily, but with no added thrill
Grade 4	Heard as loud, with an added thrill
Grade 5	Heard as loud across the entire praecordium, with a thrill
Grade 6	Audible without a stethoscope ('heard at the end of the bed')

Table 7.3 Grading the intensity of heart murmurs.

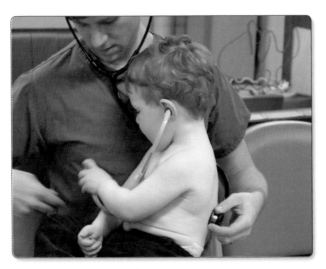

Figure 7.9 Listening to the lung bases.

Palpate for a liver edge, and discern whether the liver is enlarged. In tricuspid regurgitation, where the impulse from the right ventricle is transmitted back through the open tricuspid valve, the liver may be pulsatile.

Feel the ankles for oedema, and inspect the toenails for clubbing.

See **Table 7.4** for a summary of cardiovascular examination.

Investigations

Key cardiovascular investigations are:
- oxygen saturation
- blood pressure
- electrocardiography (ECG)

Oxygen saturation

Saturation monitors are more sensitive at picking up cyanosis than the human eye. Oxygen saturation should be checked in a child who looks unwell if the equipment is available.

General inspection	Weight, height, head (occiptofrontal) circumference Colour Respiratory rate
Hands	Pulses Fingernails (clubbing, splinters) Blood pressure
Face	Anaemia Jaundice Central cyanosis
Chest inspection	Visible impulses Scars
Chest palpation	Apex side, site Heaves, thrills
Chest auscultation	Presence of murmur Where murmur is loudest Timing of any murmur Radiation of any murmur Grade of any murmur
General	Pulmonary oedema Hepatomegaly Peripheral oedema
Investigations	Oxygen saturation ECG Blood pressure

Table 7.4 Summary of paediatric cardiovascular examination and associated investigations.

Remember that a minimum of 5 g/dL of deoxygenated blood needs to be present before cyanosis is clinically recognisable, and therefore children with anaemia may not appear blue.

Blood pressure

Measuring the blood pressure in children is technically challenging, and the result should be interpreted alongside percentile charts.

Measurement of the blood pressure requires a correctly sized cuff; the cuff should cover two-thirds of the distance between the axilla and the antecubital fossa on the upper arm. The child should (ideally) be quiet and calm.

ECG

The ECG varies throughout childhood. In the first years of life, T-wave inversion is normal in leads V1, V2 and V3; the pattern gradually changes towards an adult pattern. A specialist textbook should be consulted for more information on the paediatric ECG, but the same rules of interpretation apply as in adults. An ECG is interpreted step-wise by establishing:

- the patient's name and date of birth
- the date of the ECG
- heart rate
- heart rhythm
- axis
- P-wave morphology
- PR interval
- QRS morphology
- QT interval
- ST segment
- T-wave morphology

7.3 Clinical scenarios

A 5-year-old boy with an incidental finding of a murmur

A 5-year-old boy is brought to the emergency department with an urticarial rash that has been caused by eating a strawberry while at a friend's house. He is otherwise well, with no past medical history except for the strawberry allergy.

Examination reveals him to be mildly tachycardic, and a soft heart murmur is heard at the left lower sternal edge; the murmur does not radiate and it cannot be heard over the other valve areas. The murmur is early in systole and there is no diastolic component. There is normal splitting of the heart sounds. On being told about the murmur, the boy's mother is concerned, because he has never had a heart murmur before. Blood pressure and oxygen saturations are normal.

Differential diagnosis

- a pathological murmur, caused, for example, by an ASD, a VSD or pulmonary stenosis

- an innocent murmur, also known as a functional or benign murmur

Further information

The murmur is soft and does not radiate. The boy appears otherwise fit and well. The murmur changes with both respiration and posture. Both heart sounds are normal, and there is no abnormal fixed splitting of S2.

Concluding differential diagnosis

The boy has an innocent murmur, possibly more pronounced at present because he has a tachycardia associated with the allergic reaction. The mother is advised to take the boy to see the GP in 2 weeks, and if the murmur can be heard again then, he should be referred to a paediatric clinic.

A 9-year-old boy with a history of collapse while playing football

A 9-year-old boy is brought in to the emergency department by ambulance after he collapsed during a football match. His games teacher performed cardiopulmonary resuscitation and the boy recovered very quickly. He is now tired but says that he 'feels fine'.

Differential diagnosis

The differential diagnosis includes:

- seizure
- syncope ('fainting')
- arrhythmia
- ventricular outflow tract obstruction (e.g. aortic stenosis, coarctation of the aorta, obstructive cardiomyopathy)
- cardiomyopathy
- pericarditis

Further information

No seizure was witnessed. The boy has not been feeling unwell and he had no presyncopal symptoms such as dizziness, faintness, nausea or visual disturbance.

Examination is normal. There are no murmurs, which makes outflow tract obstruction unlikely. There is no pericardial rub, which makes pericarditis less likely. An ECG shows a corrected QT interval of 490 milliseconds; this is prolonged.

Concluding differential diagnosis

The boy has long QT syndrome, which is caused by an inherited abnormality of a membrane ion channel on the cardiac myocyte. A patient with long QT syndrome is susceptible to arrhythmias, which are most likely to occur when the heart is stressed (as during sports or swimming). Other family members should be screened and the boy should be referred to a paediatric cardiologist.

> ## Clinical insight
>
> Key points from this chapter:
> - a sick neonate may have a cardiac problem
> - always palpate the femoral arteries
> - know the anatomy – it explains the clinical presentation
> - look carefully for scars on the chest
> - think about what might be heard before using the stethoscope

The abdomen

The examination of the abdomen tends to focus on the gastrointestinal tract, but it is important to consider the urinary system and the reproductive system as well. As with all paediatric presentations, the age of the child helps to narrow the differential diagnosis and to focus the examination.

8.1 Common presentations

The key presentations of abdominal conditions include:
- abdominal pain
- vomiting
- diarrhoea

Abdominal pain

The differential diagnosis for abdominal pain can be considered in accordance with the patient's age and the symptoms associated with the pain (**Table 8.1**). Common conditions that present with abdominal pain include:
- constipation
- urinary tract infection (UTI)
- acute appendicitis

The key in taking the history is, 'When did the pain start?'.
Common causes of acute abdominal pain include:
- infection, e.g. gastroenteritis, UTI
- surgical pathology, e.g. appendicitis

Chronic causes of abdominal pain (i.e. pain lasting for longer than 2 weeks) may be due to:
- constipation
- inflammation, as in inflammatory bowel disease

One of the most important features of acute abdominal pain in children is that it may be caused by serious but non-gastrointestinal pathology.

> **Clinical insight**
>
> When a child presents with acute abdominal pain, remember the important non-abdominal causes, e.g. lower lobe pneumonia, diabetic ketoacidosis.

Approximate age	Pathology
0–2 years	Gastroenteritis UTI Intussusception Hernia
3–12 years	Gastroenteritis Constipation UTI Pneumonia Diabetic ketoacidosis Mesenteric adenitis Testicular torsion
Adolescence	Testicular pathology Acute appendicitis Ovarian disorders Trauma Pregnancy Inflammatory bowel disease

Table 8.1 Common causes of abdominal pain. Note that young children may report any pain as arising from the abdomen; therefore an ENT examination should always be performed in a febrile child with abdominal pain and no clear abdominal cause. UTI, urinary tract infection.

Constipation

Constipation is a very common cause of chronic or recurrent abdominal pain in children.

Pathology Most childhood constipation is functional, a combination of dietary factors (e.g. low-fibre diet, inadequate hydration) and psychosocial factors (e.g. a reluctance to defecate in school toilets). There are some children who have a rare cause for their constipation (e.g. Hirschsprung disease, in which there is an abnormality in the neuronal development of the intestine).

Clinical features Children with constipation may present with decreased frequency of defecation and hard pellet-like or large torpedo-like stools that are difficult to pass, often causing pain and fresh blood per rectum. Many of these children experience frequent, intermittent abdominal pain, especially when the constipation is severe.

Younger children often develop a stool-withholding pattern, crouching down to prevent their bowels opening, which can lead to a very impacted rectum. Liquid stool from above can leak out into their underwear, often causing diagnostic confusion.

Signs on examination may include a mass in the left iliac fossa that can be indented, with the texture of putty.

Urinary tract infection

UTI is a common cause of abdominal pain in children, and it is therefore imperative to test the urine in all children who present with abdominal pain. Repeated undetected UTIs can cause scarring in the kidneys, which in turn may lead to hypertension and renal failure in later life, although this is fortunately rare.

Pathology UTI can occur anywhere along the length of the urinary tract. Generally, UTIs are divided into:
- lower UTIs, e.g. cystitis
- upper UTIs, e.g. pyelonephritis

The commonest cause of UTIs are Gram-negative bacteria, especially *Escherichia coli*. Children may have anatomical abnormalities of their urinary tract that predispose them to infection, most commonly by causing vesicoureteric reflux (**Figure 8.1**).

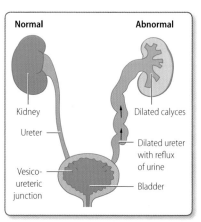

Figure 8.1 Vesicoureteric reflux.

Clinical features Some of the common symptoms of a UTI in children are:

- fever
- a non-specific feeling of being 'unwell'
- decreased appetite
- nausea and vomiting
- abdominal pain (often suprapubic or loin pain)
- dysuria and urinary frequency
- secondary nocturnal enuresis

Acute appendicitis

Acute appendicitis is the commonest surgical cause of the acute abdomen in children.

Pathology Appendicitis is caused by inflammation of the vermiform appendix.

Clinical features Children with acute appendicitis may present with abdominal pain. Classically the pain starts in the periumbilical region (as referred pain) but then spreads to the right iliac fossa when the peritoneum becomes inflamed and gives localisation to the pain. Children may also feel generally unwell with a decreased appetite, nausea and vomiting.

Vomiting

Vomiting is one of the commonest symptoms presenting to doctors who care for children. As in other areas of paediatric practice, the age of the child is intimately related to the likely causes. A good history is again the key.

The most important initial discriminator is whether the vomiting is acute (of less than 2 weeks' duration) or chronic and intermittent (of more than 2 weeks' duration).

Acute vomiting is most commonly caused by a viral infection, such as norovirus. A respiratory infection causing a cough can give rise to post-tussive vomiting.

In young children a simple fever can cause vomiting, as can almost any infection of any system. There are some key red flags to watch for:

- persisting vomiting and fever (of more than 24 hours' duration) but without diarrhoea – this can suggest bacterial meningitis

Clinical insight

Acute vomiting with fever that persists for more than 24 hours is a worrying feature, particularly if there is no diarrhoea. Consider meningitis.

- bile-stained vomitus – in such cases, bowel obstruction (e.g. from a volvulus) must be excluded

Clinical insight

A child with acute bile-stained (dark green) vomitus needs urgent surgical assessment to exclude a bowel obstruction.

Chronic or intermittent vomiting is very common, particularly in infants. Parents often worry about it, because infants frequently vomit or posset small amounts of milk after feeding. This is normal.

The causes of vomiting can be considered in three groups (**Table 8.2**):

- vomiting with a 'central' (intracranial) aetiology
- vomiting with a 'peripheral', non-gastrointestinal aetiology
- vomiting resulting from a gastrointestinal problem

Two important gastrointestinal causes of vomiting are:

- gastro-oesophageal reflux disease (GORD)
- pyloric stenosis

Gastro-oesophageal reflux disease

GORD is a common cause of regurgitation and vomiting in infants; it is less common in older children.

Pathology GORD is caused by a functionally immature gastro-oesophageal sphincter that allows stomach contents and acid to reflux into the oesophagus. Most cases occur in normal infants, but infants with a neurological disease such as cerebral palsy can have severe GORD.

Clinical features The main clinical features of GORD that may be described by parents are:

- posseting and regurgitation
- excessive crying, especially after feeds

Central causes	Typical associated features
Raised intracranial pressure	Morning headaches
Migraine	Aura, flashing lights, headache
Brainstem disease	Nystagmus, ataxia
Peripheral causes	
Otitis media	Ear pain, ear discharge
Vestibular disease	Dizziness
Diabetic ketoacidosis	Raised blood sugar
Urinary tract infection	Fever, dysuria
Pregnancy	Positive beta-hCG
Gastrointestinal causes	
Gastroenteritis	Fever, diarrhoea
Pyloric stenosis	Presents in a baby, with a palpable mass and projectile vomiting
Appendicitis	Right iliac fossa pain
Intestinal obstruction	Bile-stained vomitus

Table 8.2 Causes of vomiting in children and typical associated features. hCG, human chorionic gonadotropin.

- recurrent apnoea
- abnormal neck extension (Sandifer syndrome)

Pyloric stenosis

Pyloric stenosis is an uncommon but important cause of vomiting in infants, classically boys around the age of 4–8 weeks.

Pathology In pyloric stenosis, progressive hypertrophy of the muscle surrounding the pylorus of the stomach causes gastric outflow obstruction, resulting in the associated clinical features.

Clinical features Infants present with increasing vomiting, described as 'projectile' because the vomitus can travel a significant distance. They are eager feeders and may present with weight loss and dehydration caused by the lack of absorbed feeds.

Diarrhoea

Diarrhoeal illness is the biggest killer worldwide of children aged under 5 years. It is currently defined, by the World Health Organization, as 'having three or more loose or liquid stools per day'.

Individual patients and parents have widely different ideas as to what constitutes diarrhoea, from an increased frequency of normal motions through to the passage of persistently liquid stools.

The causes can again be thought of in terms of

- acute diarrhoea (of less than 2 weeks' duration), which is most commonly due to infective gastroenteritis or drugs
- chronic diarrhoea (of more than 2 weeks' duration), the features of which are listed in **Table 8.3**

Two important differential diagnoses of diarrhoea are:

- gastroenteritis
- inflammatory bowel disease

Gastroenteritis

Gastroenteritis is the commonest cause of acute diarrhoea in children.

Malabsorptive diarrhoea	Typical features
Coeliac disease	Poor weight gain, lethargy, pallor
Cystic fibrosis	Failure to thrive, chest infections
Post-gastroenteritis (brush border enzyme deficiency)	Follows acute infection, positive stool reducing substances
Secretory diarrhoea	
Cholera	Occurs during an epidemic, profuse watery stools
Inflammatory diarrhoea	
Inflammatory bowel disease (Crohn disease, ulcerative colitis)	Blood or mucus in stools, abdominal pain
Cow's milk protein intolerance	Rashes, atopic family history, blood in stools

Table 8.3 Causes of chronic diarrhoea in children and typical associated features.

Pathology Infectious gastroenteritis can be caused by a variety of pathogens, with viruses such as rotavirus being the most common; bacterial and protozoal causes of gastroenteritis do occur but are less common. Fresh blood in the stool may suggest a bacterial cause such as *Escherichia coli*, *Campylobacter* spp. or *Salmonella* spp., because it indicates that the child may have colitis – inflammation and bleeding of the wall of the large bowel.

Clinical features The main feature is loose stools; this term may refer to a liquid consistency of stools or to an increased frequency of defecation. Any presence of blood in the stools should be noted.

However, the most important assessment to make in a child with gastroenteritis is that of hydration. In acute severe dehydration (more than 10%), significant intravascular volume depletion occurs and leads to hypovolaemic shock.

The clinical features of dehydration constitute a spectrum of severity, ranging from mild changes, such as dry mucous membranes and slight tachycardia, through to the features of shock.

Features of severe dehydration and shock The clinical features of severe dehydration and shock are:

- looking 'unwell'
- decreased energy levels, with lethargy or decreased consciousness
- pale or mottled skin
- cool extremities
- prolonged capillary refill
- decreased urine output
- tachycardia
- tachypnoea
- low blood pressure – a late sign, very serious

> **Clinical insight**
>
> A child with diarrhoea must be assessed for features of severe dehydration. If severe dehydration is present, rapid fluid resuscitation must be commenced.

Malabsorption

The common causes of malabsorption are shown in **Table 8.3**.

Malabsorptive diarrhoea may follow an infection (post-infective diarrhoea), and may be due to a secondary lactase deficiency or cow's milk protein allergy. Treatment is a temporary withdrawal of dairy products, and using a specialised milk formula such as a casein hydrolysate, or for children over 1, a non-dairy milk such as oat milk. The malabsorption is usually transient.

Coeliac disease, a gluten allergy, must always be considered, and blood tests for anti-tissue transglutaminase antibody performed, with an intestinal biopsy considered if positive. Cystic fibrosis is suggested by the coexistence of malabsorptive stools and recurrent respiratory problems.

Cow's milk protein allergy is a common cause of chronic diarrhoea and the approach is the same as for post-infective diarrhoea.

The presence of symptoms such as blood or mucus in the stool, chronic abdominal pain, or poor weight gain may suggest inflammatory bowel disease (Crohn's or ulcerative colitis)

8.2 Abdominal examination

Examination of the abdominal system in young children can be difficult, particularly the palpation of the abdomen itself. Distraction techniques can be powerful tools, and positioning of the child is important (e.g. it may be easier if the child is lying supine on the parent's lap).

The following sequence is generally used:

1. general inspection, including height and weight
2. inspection around the bed
3. examination of the hands
4. examination of the head and neck
5. examination of the chest
6. examination of the abdomen – inspection, palpation, percussion, auscultation
7. further examination
8. investigations

General inspection

To start, stand back and inspect the overall appearance of the child, in particular assessing:

- the child's clinical state – does the child look acutely unwell?
- the child's growth and nutritional state – plot the height and weight, and calculate the body mass index if appropriate (see Chapter 4)
- any obvious signs of abdominal disease, e.g. jaundice

Around the bed

Look for clues around the bed that may indicate the type of disorder the child may be suffering from. Such clues may include:

- intravenous fluids
- nutritional supplements
- packets of crisps or sweets
- routes for enteral nutrition (e.g. a gastrostomy) or parenteral nutrition (e.g. a central line)
- vomit bowls – look at the content of these
- stoma bags

Hands

Signs of abdominal disease in the hands include:

- clubbing – seen in inflammatory bowel disease and coeliac disease
- leukonychia (pale white nails) – seen in anaemia
- koilonychia (spoon-shaped nails) – seen in iron deficiency
- pallor of the palmar creases – seen in anaemia

Head and neck

Face

Assess whether the child looks dysmorphic. Certain syndromes that cause dysmorphia are associated with gut pathology [e.g. Down syndrome (trisomy 21), duodenal atresia].

Eyes

A number of signs in the eyes can give clues to the presence of abdominal disease:

- jaundice – a yellow tinge to the sclerae (icterus) is visible when the serum bilirubin reaches approximately 40 mmol/L
- xanthelasma – abnormal lipid deposits around the eyes are seen in children with an abnormal lipid profile

- pallor of the conjunctivae – a sign of anaemia
- Kayser–Fleischer rings – blue–green rings around the iris are seen in Wilson disease as a result of abnormal copper deposits

Mouth

Approach There are a number of signs of abdominal disease to look for in the mouth. First, look at the general appearance of the mouth and jaw. Then ask the child to open the mouth and inspect inside – look at the tongue, mucosa and dentition. Finally consider if there are any abnormal odours in the breath.

Appearance There may be obvious abnormalities in the mouth and jaw (e.g. cleft lip), which may have an impact on the child's ability to feed. Inside the mouth the tongue may appear smooth (atrophic glossitis). There may also be signs of dental caries and poor dentition. Aphthous ulcers may be seen in the mucosa.

Associated conditions Specific abnormalities that may be seen in the mouth include:
- brown perioral pigmentation – associated with Peutz–Jegher syndrome (hereditary intestinal polyposis syndrome), a hereditary disorder associated with hamartomatous polyps of the gastrointestinal tract
- atrophic glossitis – associated with deficiency of iron, vitamin B12 and folate
- aphthous ulcers – seen in Crohn's disease, although they are also a normal finding
- sweet-smelling breath – a sign of diabetic ketoacidosis or liver failure (hepatic foetor)

Neck

Feel for lymphadenopathy in the cervical and axiliary areas. Marked weight loss with abdominal pain and lymphadenopathy may be due to abdominal tuberculosis. Alternatively, it may be due to lymphoma, and therefore the liver and spleen should be thoroughly examined if lymphadenopathy is detected.

Chest

Most signs of abdominal disease in the chest can be detected through inspection. Look for:

- gynaecomastia – may be a sign of chronic liver disease in boys, although adolescent gynaecomastia may also be a normal finding in boys
- spider naevi – these are visible end-arterioles; more than five spider naevi in the distribution of the superior vena cava may be associated with chronic liver disease
- centripetal obesity – this can be seen in the chest and particularly the back; it can be associated with Cushing syndrome in children on long-term corticosteroids (e.g. for inflammatory bowel disease, nephrotic syndrome)

Chest auscultation should also be performed as part of the complete examination, because a lower lobe pneumonia often presents with abdominal pain.

Abdomen

Inspection

Approach and appearance First, watch the child closely during the history taking (**Figure 8.2**): the child who presents with abdominal pain and then walks easily to the bed and climbs up on to it may not be in too much distress. Ask the child to sit up and take off his or her shirt, and watch the child's eyes for discomfort as this is done.

Is the abdomen distended? Toddlers often have a protuberant abdomen, and this must be differentiated from an abnormally distended abdomen.

Is the abdomen moving with respiration? An abdomen that is being held still and rigid may be a sign of peritonism. Ask the child to 'suck in the tummy' as far as possible, then to push it out as far as possible, then to cough. If the child cannot do these things, he or she probably has abdominal pain and may have peritonitis.

Inspect the abdomen, including in the flanks, for scars suggestive of previous surgery. It is important to expose the child down to the inguinal regions, but leave underwear on in older

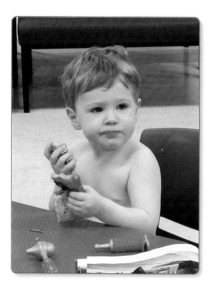

Figure 8.2 General inspection – with his relaxed demeanour and enjoyment of playing, this child probably does not have abdominal pain.

children until looking in the genital area later in the examination. Note any stomas, surgical drains or enteral feeding tubes.

Associated conditions Children who are obviously in pain when moving or whose abdomen is rigid may have an acute abdominal emergency and may be peritonitic. Many of the possible causes are listed in **Table 8.1**; in particular, consider acute surgical causes if the child shows signs of peritonism.

Palpation

Approach Ask the child to point to where the pain is worst with one finger, and then gently feel the abdomen with warm hands, starting at the point furthest away from the pain and always looking at the child's face for signs of tenderness (**Figure 8.3**).

Feel all areas of the abdomen, initially superficially, then deeper if the child allows it. Note any areas of tenderness or masses and whether any masses are smooth, irregular or indentable. A mass that can be indented is often due simply to stool.

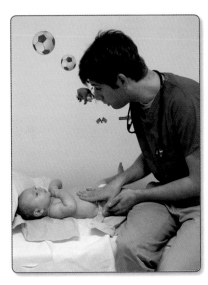

Figure 8.3 Palpating the abdomen while watching the child's eyes to see if any pain is being caused.

Feel formally for a liver and spleen. With the hand in the right iliac fossa, ask the child to breathe in and out, and gently advance the tips of your index and middle finger, holding them quite superficial, up toward the costal margin. In a neonate, 1–2 cm of liver can be felt; in a child up to 1 year of age, it is normal to be able to feel up to 1 cm of liver.

To feel for the spleen, use the same technique as for the liver, moving the fingers from the right iliac fossa to the left hypochondrium.

Feel for enlarged kidneys using ballottement. Place one hand behind the child at the costophrenic angle and attempt to lift the kidney to touch your other hand, placed on the anterior of the abdomen in the same region. A palpable kidney is generally an enlarged kidney, although a normal-sized kidney may be able to be felt in a thin child.

Associated conditions Tenderness in the abdomen has a wide differential diagnosis. The list of possible causes can be made more focused by considering the area in which the pain is worst, but in children pain and tenderness may be felt in unusual areas – for example, a young child with tonsillitis may complain of abdominal pain.

The various causes of an enlarged liver, spleen and kidneys are listed below.

Causes of hepatomegaly Key causes to exclude are:
- infectious conditions, e.g. hepatitis A infection, infectious mononucleosis
- neoplasia, e.g. leukaemia, lymphoma
- haematological disease, e.g. thalassaemia major

A palpable liver may have been pushed inferiorly by hyperexpanded lungs (e.g. in an infant with bronchiolitis). Percussion is required to confirm enlargement of the liver.

Causes of splenomegaly Key causes to exclude are:
- haematological disease, e.g. acute leukaemia, thalassaemia major
- infectious conditions, e.g. infectious mononucleosis, malaria
- vascular disease, e.g. portal hypertension secondary to chronic liver disease

Causes of enlarged kidneys Key causes to exclude are:
- polycystic kidney disease, which may be autosomal-recessive or autosomal-dominant
- nephroblastoma (Wilm tumour)

Percussion

Approach Percuss any masses to elicit whether they contain gas (in which case the percussion note will be resonant) or are solid (in which case the percussion note will be dull).

Assess for shifting dullness, the presence of which indicates ascites. With the child on the back, ascitic fluid should fall to the flanks, the central abdomen will be resonant to percussion (due to gas-containing bowel floating on the fluid) and the flanks will be dull. Then ask the child to turn on to the left side and wait for a minute, then percuss again over the central area that was previously resonant. If it is now dull then fluid has shifted to the new position and ascites is present.

Associated conditions Ascites is uncommon in children. The main causes are:

- chronic liver disease
- nephrotic syndrome
- kwashiorkor

Auscultation

Listen for bowel sounds (**Figure 8.4**), and note their presence and quality. High-pitched, tinkling, overactive sounds are indicative of distal obstruction. Absent bowel sounds – after listening for 60 seconds – suggest an ileus.

Listen over any masses and over the kidneys for bruits.

Further examination

There are a number of other things which may need to be done to complete the examination of the abdominal system:

- look in the groins (**Figure 8.5**) to assess whether there any evidence of an inguinal hernia

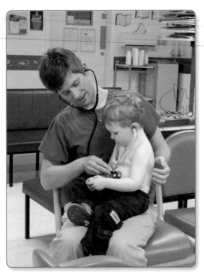

Figure 8.4 Auscultating for bowel sounds. Ideally, a child should be examined lying down but this may not be possible.

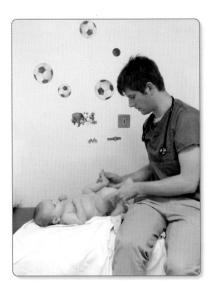

Figure 8.5 Checking the groin for hernias.

- examine the external genitalia, if indicated; it is important to examine for testicular torsion in boys who present with abdominal pain
- examine for evidence of nappy rash or thrush, if appropriate
- look at the back and the base of spine; spina bifida is a cause of constipation
- look at the lower limbs for erythema nodosum, which is associated with inflammatory bowel disease

A rectal examination should be performed only by the doctor who is going to make a decision based upon the findings, and it should be done only when clearly indicated.

See **Table 8.4** for a summary of abdominal examination.

Investigations

After the examination of the gastrointestinal system has been completed, there are a number of investigations that should be considered.

A dipstick urine test should be done to look for blood, protein, glucose, bilirubin, leukocytes and nitrites in the urine.

Component of the examination	Assessment
General inspection	Is the child well or unwell? Is the child in pain? Height and weight
Around the bed	Specialist feeds, vomit bowls
Hands	Clubbing, nails, palmar erythema
Face	Eyes, tongue, dentition, breath, mouth ulcers
Chest	Gynaecomastia, obesity
Abdomen	Scars, masses, distension, fluid, stomas
Other	Groins, back, legs
Investigations	Urine dipstick; urine microscopy; stool virology, culture and biochemistry

Table 8.4 The paediatric abdominal examination.

A positive result for leukocytes and nitrites suggests a UTI, although negative results do not exclude a UTI in infants and young children, and a urine sample must still be sent for culture.

Further tests should be considered as part of the management plan (e.g. capillary blood glucose, laboratory blood testing, imaging). However, abdominal radiographs should not be routinely considered in the work-up of a patient with abdominal pain, although abdominal ultrasound is an excellent tool for imaging the abdominal contents and it may be invaluable in conditions such as intussusception.

8.3 Clinical scenarios

A 15-year-old girl with abdominal pain

A 15-year-old girl comes to the emergency department with her parents. She has a 1-day history of severe abdominal pain. She has vomited once and had a loose stool yesterday; today she has not opened her bowels. She looks pale and has a mildly raised heart rate. She is unable to sit up on the trolley.

Differential diagnosis

The following conditions should be considered:

- gastroenteritis
- appendicitis
- ectopic pregnancy
- intestinal obstruction

Further information

Examination reveals a tender right iliac fossa with guarding, and bowel sounds are absent. She has just finished her menstrual period, and she has a regular menstrual cycle. A urinary pregnancy beta-human chorionic gonadotropin (hCG) test is negative. She has no fever and the vomitus was not bile-stained.

Concluding differential diagnosis

Although many of the differential diagnoses above are still possible, appendicitis now seems the most likely cause. The specific tenderness in the right iliac fossa is not typical of gastroenteritis, and the recent period and negative urinary hCG test make ectopic pregnancy highly unlikely. There is no bile-stained vomitus to suggest a bowel obstruction. Appendicitis is the most common of the remaining differential diagnoses, and it fits the clinical picture. Appendicitis is a clinical diagnosis and a surgical opinion should be sought.

A 3-year-old boy with chronic diarrhoea

A 3-year-old boy is brought to the GP by his mother. She is concerned because his stools always seem to be loose compared with those of other children. His mother also thinks that he has not put on much weight recently.

Differential diagnosis

The following differential diagnoses should be considered:

- coeliac disease
- cystic fibrosis
- lactose intolerance
- inflammatory bowel disease
- toddler diarrhoea

Further Information

On further questioning, it transpires that the diarrhoea has been present for over a year now. The stools are also foul smelling and difficult to flush away. His mother also mentions that he has had more than 10 respiratory infections in the past year. On examination, the boy is noted to be thin and he looks miserable. His records reveal a static weight, and his height velocity is now also slowing down.

Concluding differential diagnosis

The clinical features suggest malabsorption as the cause for both the diarrhoea and the failure to gain weight. Toddler diarrhoea would not lead to the growth problems. Inflammatory bowel disease is possible but unlikely in this young age group. Lactose intolerance tends to be a temporary phenomenon after an episode of acute gastroenteritis, and it only rarely causes prolonged malabsorption.

Coeliac disease and cystic fibrosis seem to be the most likely causes, and given the high number of respiratory infections that the boy has had, cystic fibrosis must be excluded.

Clinical insight

Key points from this chapter:
- abdominal pain is common, and the history is key to making a diagnosis
- look out for the danger signs of dehydration with diarrhoea or vomiting in children
- test the urine by dipstick

The nervous system

There is a close relationship between the developmental assessment and the neurological examination. In younger children the two are carried out simultaneously. (See Chapter 5 for details of the developmental assessment; some points from that chapter are repeated here.) The key to diagnosing neurological problems in children is to use the presenting symptoms and signs to determine where in the nervous system the problem is located.

9.1 Common presentations

Key presentations of neurological conditions in children include:
- headache
- weakness
- unsteady gait
- hypotonia
- hypertonia
- seizures

Headache

Differential diagnoses

Causes of headache include:
- migraine
- tension headache
- intracranial tumour

Migraine

Clinical features In some patients, migraines begin with a prodrome (a period of lethargy or restlessness). This may be followed by an aura (abnormal sensations of taste or vision, such as seeing flashing lights). The headaches are usually frontal or unilateral, and they may be throbbing or pulsating in nature.

Associated symptoms include nausea, vomiting and sensitivity to light (photophobia). The headache may last for hours or days. Sufferers are usually in late childhood or adolescence, but migraine can occur much earlier when the classical features are often not present.

If there are any focal neurological symptoms, such as limb weakness, a magnetic resonance imaging (MRI) and magnetic resonance angiography (MRA) of the brain are required to exclude an arteriovenous malformation (AVM).

Tension headache

Clinical features Tension headaches are usually bilateral, and may be associated with neck stiffness or aching neck muscles. They are much commoner than migraines, and they can be differentiated from migraines in that there are no associated features such as vomiting or visual disturbances. A tension headache can be associated with triggers, such as long periods spent in front of a bright screen (e.g. a computer or television screen) or prolonged squinting.

> **Clinical insight**
>
> Children suffering from tension headaches should have their vision checked – they may simply need corrective spectacles.

Intracranial tumour

Clinical features Tumours inside the skull (space-occupying lesions) cause symptoms as a result of:
- increased pressure inside the skull
- a mass effect on structures adjacent to the tumour

Raised intracranial pressure The symptoms of raised intracranial pressures are headaches, nausea and vomiting, predominantly in the morning. Late signs include raised blood pressure and a slow pulse (the Cushing reflex). There may be visual disturbance when pressure is raised around the optic nerve.

> **Clinical insight**
>
> In children who present with headaches that wake them during the night or that are present first thing in the morning, a brain MRI should be considered to exclude an intracranial lesion.

Effects on adjacent structures The effects of the tumour on adjacent structures result in symptoms and signs related to the function of the affected area of the brain. For example, a tumour in the occipital lobe will cause visual disturbances or blindness. A parietal lobe tumour may cause abnormal sensations or weakness. As a tumour grows in size, the signs and symptoms will become more severe, and other associated symptoms, such as seizures, may develop.

Weakness

Weakness can be caused by any insult to a structure between the central nervous system (CNS) and the effector organ, the muscle (**Figure 9.1**). It is helpful when considering the differential diagnosis to establish whether the weakness is acute (**Table 9.1**) or chronic (**Table 9.2**) in onset.

Differential diagnoses

Central aetiology:
- stroke
- acute disseminated encephalomyelitis

Peripheral aetiology:
- poliomyelitis

Muscular aetiology:
- muscular dystrophy

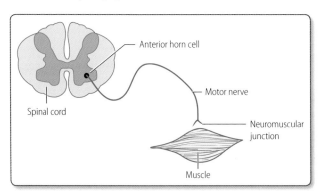

Figure 9.1 The neuromuscular pathway.

Central causes	Peripheral causes
Stroke	Nerve root compression
Intracranial lesion	Anterior Horn cell infection (poliomyelitis)
Intracranial infection	Peripheral neuropathy, e.g. Guillain–Barré syndrome
Demyelination	Neuromuscular paralysis, e.g. botulism, neuromuscular blocking drugs Acute myositis

Table 9.1 Key central and peripheral causes of acute weakness.

Central causes	Peripheral causes
Cerebral palsy	Nerve root compression
Intracranial lesion	Anterior horn cell disease, e.g. spinal muscular atrophy
Demyelination	Peripheral neuropathy Myasthenia gravis Muscular dystrophy

Table 9.2 Key central and peripheral causes of chronic weakness.

Stroke

Pathology A stroke occurs when the arterial blood supply to an area of cerebral cortex is suddenly stopped, resulting in the death of neurones dependent on the affected artery. A stroke can be haemorrhagic (e.g. caused by rupture of an aneurysm) or thrombotic (arterial or venous thrombosis).

Unlike in adults, atherosclerotic thrombosis is rare in children, and if thrombosis occurs it is likely that there is either an underlying prothrombotic state or an abnormal blood vessel (e.g. narrowing of a vessel following an infection such as chickenpox). If the red cells are abnormal, as in sickle cell disease, stroke may occur as a result of vessel occlusion.

Clinical features The signs and symptoms depend on the area of brain tissue affected. For example, if the middle cerebral artery is affected, then weakness may be a feature.

Newborn babies may have seizures following a stroke.

Acute disseminated encephalomyelitis

Pathology Acute disseminated encephalomyelitis is an immune-mediated destruction of the myelin sheath of neurones, usually following a viral illness. It is particularly associated with measles.

Clinical features Presentation is usually 2–3 weeks after a viral infection with weakness and features of encephalopathy (decreased consciousness and seizures).

Poliomyelitis

Pathology Poliovirus infection affects the anterior horn cells of the spinal cord.

Clinical features The clinical features are lower motor neurone signs of weakness and absent reflexes. The signs may be bilateral or, more commonly, unilateral.

Muscular dystrophy

Pathology In muscular dystrophy, dystrophic ('abnormally grown') muscle fibres arise as a result of a genetic abnormality.

Clinical features The muscle functions abnormally, and the patient suffers from chronic weakness in the skeletal muscles. Affected children walk later than their peers, and they may present with developmental delay.

Unsteady gait

Unsteadiness of gait may be due to:
- an ataxic gait
- a hemiplegic gait

Ataxic gait

Clinical features An ataxic gait is broad-based (with the feet held wide apart) and stumbling. It occurs as a result of cerebellar dysfunction.

Hemiplegic gait

Clinical features A hemiplegic gait is a stiff-legged gait in which the affected leg has increased tone and is held with the toe pointing down. The stiff leg has to swing outwards and is brought round in a semicircle during walking.

Hypotonia

Hypotonia is decreased tone or floppiness. Decreased tone may be associated with weakness, and the differential diagnoses of the two overlap.

Differential diagnoses

There are many possible causes of hypotonia (**Table 9.3**). Important differential diagnoses include:
- a chromosomal abnormality, e.g. Down syndrome (trisomy 21)
- a genetic abnormality, e.g. spinal muscular atrophy

Central causes	Peripheral causes	Generalised causes
Genetic syndromes, e.g. Down syndrome	Spinal cord disease, e.g. anterior horn cell disease, such as spinal msuscular atrophy, poliomyelitis	Inborn errors of metabolism, e.g. aminoacidurias
Cerebral palsy (numerous causes, e.g. infection, trauma, ischaemic encephalopathy)	Neuromuscular junction disorders, e.g. myasthenia gravis	Endocrine causes, e.g. hypothyroidism
	Muscular disease, e.g. muscular dystrophy, congenital myopathy, mitochondrial disorders	
	Peripheral nervous system disease, e.g. hereditary sensory neuropathy	

Table 9.3 Common causes of hypotonia.

Down syndrome

Pathology Down syndrome results from excess copies of the genes of chromosome 21 in the genome, most often three complete copies of the chromosome (trisomy 21).

Clinical features For a full description of Down syndrome, see Chapter 15. Hypotonia is commonly found in neonates with trisomy 21.

Spinal muscular atrophy

Pathology Spinal muscular atrophy is a genetic abnormality that results in degeneration of neurones in the anterior spinal cord, resulting in decreased skeletal muscle power.

Clinical features Children with spinal muscular atrophy may present in the neonatal period or in the first few months of life as being hypotonic, or they present at 6–9 months when they are noted to be missing motor milestones, e.g. not sitting or rolling. Assessment of this condition therefore demonstrates how the neurological and developmental examinations overlap.

Hypertonia

Hypertonia is increased tone, or spasticity. The affected region (which may be a limb or the trunk) is held stiff, and it is difficult to move it passively on examination. Hypertonia occurs when there is damage to the CNS – an upper motor neurone lesion.

Differential diagnoses

Key causes of hypertonia are
- cerebral palsy
- stroke

Cerebral palsy

Pathology Cerebral palsy is defined as a 'fixed insult to the developing brain'. The common causes are:
- genetic abnormality
- hypoxic-ischaemic brain injury

- intraventricular haemorrhage (which may occur in premature neonates)
- infection, e.g. meningitis
- trauma from a head injury

Clinical features The pattern of signs depends on the site of the injury and the developing abilities of the child.

For example, children with intraventricular haemorrhages often have motor problems (weakness and spasticity) because the site of the bleeding often involves the basal ganglia (which act as motor relays in the midbrain).

A widespread brain injury, such as might occur following hypoxic ischaemic encephalopathy, may affect multiple brain functions. Children with such injuries may have problems with movements, sight, hearing, swallowing and oesophageal motility (and therefore be at risk of aspiration and pneumonia) and continence.

Stroke

Pathology A stroke causes hypertonia because the upper motor neurone lesion prevents inhibitory signals descending from the cerebral cortex to the spinal cord. As a result, the muscles are held contracted.

Clinical features Clinical features of stroke are:
- hypertonia and weakness in the affected limb or limbs
- exaggerated tendon reflexes (again, as a result of the loss of descending inhibition from the CNS)

Seizures

Seizures are the result of a chaotic discharge of electricity in the brain. They may be generalised (affecting the whole body) or focal (affecting just one part of the body).

Differential diagnoses

Seizures may be the presentation of:
- a febrile convulsion
- epilepsy

- an acute insult to the brain, which may be due to infection, trauma, tumour or hypoglyceamia

Febrile convulsions

Pathology A febrile convulsion is a seizure that occurs either before or during a period of pyrexia. The cause is unknown, although there is often a family history of febrile convulsions.

Clinical features Febrile convulsions occur between the ages of 6 months and 6 years. They are usually short and generalised (the child loses consciousness and shakes all four limbs) and are followed by a postictal phase of drowsiness. These features help to differentiate a febrile convulsion from rigors, in which a febrile child shivers but does not lose consciousness or have a seizure.

Epilepsy

Pathology In epilepsy a person has repeated seizures. Epilepsy may occur following an insult to the brain (e.g. children with cerebral palsy may suffer from epilepsy), or it may have no clear cause.

Clinical features Seizures may be focal or generalised. Focal seizures affect one area of the body; there may be lip smacking, a repeated spasm of the hand or a brief moment of vacant staring (an absence seizure).

Generalised seizures affect the whole body. The child may collapse and start to shake uncontrollably. The majority of generalised seizures are short in duration and self-limiting; however, drug therapy may be required to stop the seizure if it lasts for more than 5 minutes. There may be tongue biting or urinary incontinence, although these can also occur secondary to a faint (syncope).

Acute insult to the brain

Pathology If the electrochemical homoeostasis of the brain is disturbed, there may be uncoordinated electrical discharges, resulting in seizures.

Causes include:
- infections, e.g. meningitis, encephalitis
- trauma, which can produce diffuse axonal injury or intra-cranial bleeding
- tumours, which can act as an electrical focus for seizures
- hypoglycaemia

Clinical features Clinical features depend on the acute insult. Trauma or infection may be subtle or very obvious.

9.2 Neurological examination

The neurological examination of the child consists essentially of the following components, which are usually attempted in the listed order below. However, in young children and infants, order does not work well, and as with other aspects of clinical examination in this age group, you must do what you can when you can. Observation forms the major component of the examination.

A suggested sequence for the neurological examination is:
- general assessment of the child, including mental status
- gait, if the child is ambulant
- head, face and cranial nerves
- limbs
  - tone
  - power and muscle function
  - co-ordination and movements
  - tendon reflexes
  - sensation
- cerebellar signs
- primitive and protective reflexes (in infants)

There is a close relationship and commonality between the developmental assessment and the neurological examination, and indeed for younger children they are done simultaneously. (See Chapter 5 for details of the developmental assessment; some points from that chapter are repeated here.)

This section concentrates on the neurological examination in younger children; for older children the examination follows the same pattern as for an adult.

General assessment

The general assessment of a child at the beginning of a neurological assessment should include:

- general appearance
- mental status
- the skin, looking for neurocutaneous markers

In order to do this general assessment properly, is it important that the child should be appropriately exposed – for a full neurological examination the child should be undressed to the underwear.

General appearance

Observe whether there are any obvious clues to underlying neurological disease. The presence of an object that helps a child to function is a clue to an underlying disability, e.g. a gastrostomy tube suggests possible unsafe swallowing. Clues may include:

- a wheelchair
- hearing aids
- feeding or gastrostomy tubes
- splints supporting the ankles, which are used in hypertonia
- abnormal posture, which may be extensor and spastic or hypotonic and floppy
- lack of visual alertness, i.e. lack of fixed gaze on objects or people's faces
- use of nappies beyond the expected age

Mental status

Definition Mental status can be considered synonymous with 'level of consciousness'. It describes how alert a child is.

Approach If a child appears drowsy or unconscious, and you are concerned, it is appropriate to firmly rub the child on the sternum with a finger or knuckle. This provides a painful central stimulus. If the child opens the eyes, vocalises to the pain or moves, then the level of consciousness can be assessed. If a sternal rub is not possible (e.g. because of sternal injury), then a squeeze of the trapezius muscle or pressure to the superior orbit may be applied.

Appearance If the brain is impaired, it will 'switch off' its functions in a predictable fashion. There are three areas of brain function to be considered:

- speech
- eye opening
- motor response

These three areas are used to make up the components of the Glasgow Coma Scale (**Table 9.4**). This scoring system was initially developed for assessing adults with head injuries, but it has been adapted for children.

Associated conditions A decreased score on the Glasgow Coma Scale is associated with a global insult or an injury that affects the whole brain. Examples of such injuries are:

- low blood pressure, e.g. in sepsis or haemorrhage
- infection affecting the whole brain, e.g. in encephalitis
- diffuse axonal injury, e.g. following a traumatic injury to the head

Skin (neurocutaneous markers)

Definition Neurocutaneous markers are specific lesions or appearances of the skin that are associated with neurological disease.

Approach Some neurocutaneous markers may be obvious, such as a port-wine stain or a large neurofibroma. These lesions may be brought to the doctor's attention by parents. Other markers, such as café-au-lait spots or ash-leaf macules, may be more subtle and should be sought if the condition in which they are found is suspected.

Appearance There is a wide variety of neurocutaneous markers. Some examples and their associated conditions are listed in **Table 9.5**.

	Infants	Children	Score
Eye opening	Open spontaneously	Open spontaneously	4
	Open in response to verbal stimuli	Open in response to verbal stimuli	3
	Open in response to pain only	Open in response to pain only	2
	No response	No response	1
Verbal response	Coos and babbles	Oriented, appropriate	5
	Irritable cries	Confused	4
	Cries in response to pain	Inappropriate words	3
	Moans in response to pain	Incomprehensible words or non-specific sounds	2
	No response	No response	1
Motor response	Moves spontaneously and purposefully	Obeys commands	6
	Withdraws to touch	Localises painful stimulus	5
	Withdraws in response to pain	Withdraws in response to pain	4
	Responds to pain with decorticate posturing (abnormal flexion)	Responds to pain with flexion	3
	Responds to pain with decerebrate posturing (abnormal extension)	Responds to pain with extension	2
	No response	No response	1

Table 9.4 The Glasgow Coma Scale in infants and children. The three values from each test are considered separately and as a total in assessing mental state.

Gait

The way in which a child walks can give clues to the presence and possible site of a neurological problem. The appearance and clinical features of two gaits – a hemiplegic gait and an ataxic gait – that arise from CNS pathologies have been considered above.

Name	Appearance	Associated conditions
Café-au-lait spot	Large, flat freckles	Numerous conditions, including neurofibromatosis
Port-wine stain	Purple-red birthmark across the face	Sturge–Weber syndrome
Ash leaf macule	Ash-leaf shaped flat area of depigmentation, often over the sacrum	Tuberous sclerosis

Table 9.5 Neurocutaneous markers, their appearance and associated conditions.

The assessment of some features of gait disturbance overlap with the musculoskeletal examination, and it is important to consider and assess the developmental level when looking at how a child walks.

In the assessment of gait it is important to consider:
- lower limb appearance, tone and muscle bulk
- walking, turning and balance
- hopping, skipping and running

Lower limb appearance and leg length

Approach Inspect the lower limbs and look at their shape to assess if they are symmetrical. Look for any obvious abnormality, scars, and splints or supports. Assess the muscle size and tone, and look for abnormal movements. These assessments can also be done if the child is in a wheelchair.

Appearance Unilateral lower limb neurological disease may be obvious on inspection; in poliomyelitis, for example, one limb has pronounced muscle wasting. If the tone is raised in one leg then the foot may be held with the toe on the ground and the foot pointing down. Muscle bulk may be increased in one muscle group.

Associated conditions Hypertonia is associated with a CNS injury, e.g. cerebral palsy or stroke. Muscle hypertrophy in the lower limbs – specifically in the gastrocnemius and soleus muscles – is found in muscular dystrophy.

Walking, turning and balance

Approach Ask the child if he or she can walk – the answer to this question may be obvious if you have seen the child walk in, but a child who is in a wheelchair may nevertheless be able to walk a few steps with help.

Ask the child to walk away from you and observe the gait from behind. Ask the child to take a few steps, then to stop, to turn around and to walk back. If there is a balance problem it may become obvious when the child is turning. A child who is old enough should be asked to heel–toe walk.

Appearance Gait abnormalities include a pronounced 'toe-stepping' gait, a broad-based gait and unilateral or bilateral abnormalities in which the feet do not lift from the floor but instead sweep around in a semicircle.

Associated conditions Associated conditions should be looked for:
- 'toe-stepping' may be habitual and non-pathological in younger children (aged 3–5 years), or it may be the result of hypertonia in the leg
- a broad-based gait may be due to imbalance (as a result of either cerebellar or middle-ear disease)
- a sweeping gait may be caused by hypertonia secondary to a CNS injury.

Hopping, skipping, running

Approach The abilities to hop, skip and run are associated with motor development and should be tested to assess whether a child is meeting the expected developmental milestones (see Chapter 5).

Head, face and cranial nerves

The skull contains the brain, and developmental problems of the skull may therefore affect brain development. Some chro-

mosomal or genetic abnormalities that can affect neurodevelopment may be associated with an abnormal facial appearance. Neurological examination of the head therefore includes:
- the skull
- the face
- the cranial nerves

Skull

Figure 9.2 shows the sutures and fontanelles of the infant skull.

Approach First, using a tape measure, measure the maximum occipitofrontal circumference (OFC). Do this three times and take the average. Plot it on a centile chart.

Then:
- check whether the anterior fontanelle is open or closed (**Figure 9.3**) and whether it is bulging or sunken
- feel along the skull sutures for any abnormalities (early or late fusion, ridges or abnormal shapes)
- auscultate the side of the head for intracranial bruits (an audible 'whooshing' of blood, similar in sound to that of a cardiac murmur)

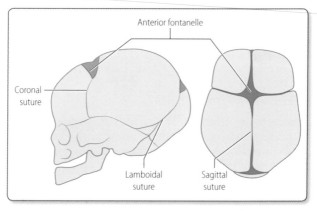

Figure 9.2 Skull sutures and the anterior and posterior fontanelles.

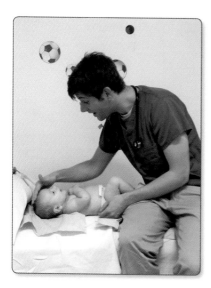

Figure 9.3 Feeling for the anterior fontanelle.

Appearance A very small head may suggest microcephaly, but beware that it can be perfectly normal to have a small head. Microcephaly is defined as an OFC below the 0.4th centile. Some causes of microcephaly are shown in **Table 9.6**.

A large head may similarly be normal, often with a family history. Macrocephaly is defined as an OFC above the 99.6th centile. Some causes of macrocephaly are shown in **Table 9.6**. There may be flattening of one side of the skull (plagiocephaly), which may be:

- benign deformational plagiocephaly, a simple mechanical issue arising from the child lying on one side of the head
- craniosynostosis (premature closure of one or other of the sutures)

Associated conditions The commonest forms of craniosynostosis (see **Figure 9.2**) are:

- sagittal synostosis – premature fusion of the saggital suture
- coronal synostosis – premature fusion of the coronal suture

Microcephaly	Macrocephaly
Genetic syndromes	Hydrocephalus
Prenatal infection	Fragile X
Prenatal ischaemia	Overgrowth conditions, e.g. Beckwith syndrome
Craniosynostosis (premature fusion of the sutures)	

Table 9.6 Causes of abnormal head size.

If coronal synostosis is bilateral, the head cannot grow in the anterior–posterior direction and so it grows upwards. The resulting head shape is called turricephaly. If coronal synostosis is unilateral, the head grows asymmetrically (plagiocephaly).

In saggital synostosis, the head cannot grow in the perpendicular plane. It therefore grows to be narrow and elongated, which is called scaphocephaly.

Intracranial bruit Auscultate each side of the head in children who have a history of headaches or when there has been a suggestion of sudden loss of power or sensation on one side. There may be an arterio-venous malformation (AVM) – an abnormal connection between arteries and veins inside the skull. AVMs can leak, causing headache, weakness or abnormal sensation.

Face

Approach The following points should be assessed:
- does the child have an abnormal facial appearance (dysmorphism)?
- does the child look like anyone else in the family?
- is there apparent asymmetry or weakness of the face?
- is one side of the face bigger than the other?
- is the upper eyelid drooping and obscuring the pupil (ptosis)?

Appearance If a child is dysmorphic, it is important to be able to describe the individual features that make up the dysmorphism. For example, in Noonan syndrome (see Chapter 15), the eyes may have an abnormal appearance:

- the eyes are far apart (hypertelorism)
- the eyelids droop (bilateral ptosis)
- the fold of skin at the inner aspect of the eye is bigger than would be usual in a Caucasian (prominent epicanthic folds)

Reference textbooks of paediatrics have tables for these features and terms; it is an extensive list.

Associated conditions Facial appearance may suggest a local pathology, such as a cranial nerve problem, a genetic problem or a syndromic diagnosis.

Cranial nerve examination

In fully co-operative older children, the same approach to cranial nerve examination is used as in adult patients. In younger children, this aspect of the neurological examination requires a more pragmatic approach. Most of the assessment is gleaned from simple observation. Each nerve is considered in turn.

CN I (olfactory nerve) Ask the child if he or she has noticed any change in the sense of smell. This may be formally tested using standard odours, but it is not normally tested in routine practice unless there has been significant mid-facial trauma.

CN II (optic nerve) Check for visual responsiveness. Young infants should fix and follow by 6–8 weeks of age.

Red reflex Look for the red reflex by shining an ophthalmoscope into the eye and looking for the red reflection of the retina. A white reflex is very concerning and may suggest serious retinal disease, such as retinoblastoma. A lack of the red reflex may be picked up incidentally when a photograph reveals a white reflex in a child's eye.

Reflex afferent papillary defect Check the pupils for responses to light, including for a reflex afferent pupillary defect (RAPD).

When a light is shone into one of the pupils, that pupil constricts via the direct light reflex. This happens because the light is transmitted via CN II (the afferent pathway) and then pupillary constriction occurs via the parasympathetic branch within CN III (the efferent pathway). At the same time, the opposite pupil also constricts, the consensual light reflex, as a result of the efferent pathway being activated on the opposite side.

When a light is swung from eye to eye, the pupil into which the light is being shone should constrict, and the other pupil should also momentarily constrict before dilating.

The RAPD is a very important abnormality because it suggests there is a neurological deficit on the afferent side, such as a CN II disorder. When a light is shone into the affected eye, the eye does not constrict, and because there is less light transmitted through the affected optic nerve, the consensual reflex also fails. As the light is shone into the unaffected eye, it constricts and the consensual reflex also causes constriction of the affected eye.

Visual fields Visual field testing in a young child is very difficult. It is worth trying a technique whereby the child is distracted by something interesting being held in the central field of vision. Then, a more interesting object is slowly brought into the peripheral fields of vision, to ascertain if the child moves the gaze towards this second object.

Visual acuity Assessing visual acuity in young children is equally problematic. A young child cannot read and therefore cannot co-operate with a Snellen chart. If the child is old enough to have started reading, then check each eye in turn (covering up the other one) to check crudely whether vision is maintained.

Fundoscopy Fundoscopy is difficult in a very young child, and if there is concern about the optic nerve, then it is best practice to dilate the pupils using a mydriatic agent and arrange for an ophthalmologist to review the optic discs.

CN III (oculomotor nerve) A CN III palsy causes a dilated pupil. Look at the eye movements, because there may be a divergent squint and a ptosis on the affected side. A parent, or a toy being held up, might persuade the child to look to the side so that any divergent squint can be detected. Sometimes the child tries to compensate for a squint and the resultant diplopia by tilting the head.

CN IV (trochlear nerve) and CN VI (abducens nerve) CN IV and CN VI are best assessed by observation – for example, a young child with a CN IV or CN VI palsy may not follow a finger or an object.

Look for any paralytic strabismus, such as when one eye constantly looks outwards (the lateral gaze palsy). This indicates a CN VI palsy; it is a highly worrying sign and suggests an intracranial lesion.

CN V (trigeminal nerve) CN V function is very hard to assess in a young child. Formally assessing sensation may not be possible, and elicitation of the corneal reflex should not be attempted in a child. A parent may report slow or weak chewing if there is a problem with the motor branch of the CN V, which innervates the masseter, temporalis and pterygoid muscles.

CN VII (facial nerve) Look for facial weakness. CN VII is one of the more easily assessed cranial nerves, for weakness is apparent just by observation and by asking the child to smile (**Figure 9.4**).

CN VII palsy Upper motor neurone CN VII palsy is rare, but it may be caused by a supranuclear lesion such as a stroke or a hemispheric lesion. Congenital CN VII palsy occurs in Moebius syndrome, which is very rare.

Acute lower motor neurone CN VII palsy is common in children but rare in infants and toddlers. See **Table 9.7** for a list of causes.

It is vital that all causes of CN VII palsy should be considered. Lyme disease is a common cause and needs to be ruled out, because the facial palsy of Lyme disease may resolve without treatment and the opportunity for correct diagnosis may therefore be lost until much later, more serious complications present. If there is any possibility that the child may have been in a Lyme-endemic area in recent months, even if there is no clear history of a tick bite (as often there is not), then Lyme serology and PCR must be done.

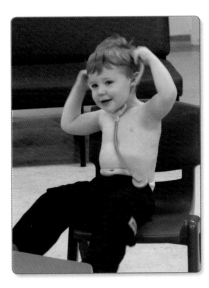

Figure 9.4 Normal CN VII nerve function: smiling and lifting the eyebrows.

Idiopathic (Bell palsy)
Herpes infection
Trauma
Vascular lesions
Hypertension
Brainstem lesions
Lyme disease

Table 9.7 Common causes of acute CN VII palsy.

CN VIII (vestibulocochlear nerve) In a young child, abnormalities of CN VIII can be suspected only from a history of symptoms of dizziness or deafness, or both.

CN IX (glossopharyngeal nerve) and CN X (vagus nerve) Inspect the mouth, and watch the movement of the uvula. It deviates towards the side of a lesion, as tone is lost in the palate. The history may suggest a problem such as a bulbar palsy, and there may be a history of feeding difficulty, choking or nasal regurgitation, as seen in conditions such as spastic cerebral palsy.

CN XI (accessory nerve) Check the sternocleidomastoid muscle, which turns the head to the opposite side. Assess the trapezius muscle, which shrugs the shoulder.

CN XII (hypoglossal nerve) Ask or encourage the child to stick the tongue out – mimicry may be required. Look for deviation to one side and fasciculations of the tongue.

Examination of the limbs

Examination of the limbs follows the usual scheme:
1. tone
2. power and muscle function
3. co-ordination and movements
4. tendon reflexes
5. sensation

Tone

Definition Tone depends on basal or 'tonic' muscle contraction. It reflects the proportion of neuromuscular junctions that are actively transmitting acetylcholine, causing muscle to contract. In healthy muscle, tone is regulated by descending inhibition from the CNS. Some muscles are maintained in an 'on' state (e.g. sphincter muscles) and relax under conscious or unconscious control. Most striated skeletal muscle is relaxed in normal circumstances, depending on a child's posture.

If there is a CNS injury, then the tone to the muscles controlled by that region of the CNS will increase, because descending inhibition is lost. This results in a stiff or spastic muscle (hypertonia).

If there is an injury to a peripheral nerve innervating a muscle, then no impulses can reach the neuromuscular junction, and the muscle fibres is not activated. This results in a floppy, weak muscle (hypotonia). Occasionally with a lower motor neurone injury, as the acetylcholine receptors migrate away from the neuromuscular junction in an attempt to find a new stimulating nerve end-plate, there are weak, uncoordinated contractions of muscle fibres, known as fasciculations.

Approach In an infant, look at the posture. A very floppy baby may lie with the limbs flat against the cot surface, the 'frog-leg' posture. A stiff baby may hold the neck hyperextended and may have the knees flexed and hands in a closed fist, with the thumb held inwards against the palm.

Bring the child from the supine to the sitting position (pull to sit) by grasping the hands, and watch for the head position. Normal infants will bring the head up quickly to a position in line with the trunk by around 3–4 months of age (**Figure 9.5**). Any significant lag of the head behind the body after the age of 4 months suggests hypotonia.

Gently hold the limbs and flex and extend the main joints. A stiff or hypertonic limb offers resistance as the joint is flexed and extended.

Check for clonus (rhythmic, beating contractions) by holding the leg and, with the other hand, rapidly dorsiflexing the relaxed ankle. Clonus may be seen and felt in the calf muscles if there is hypertonia.

Appearance

Hypotonia The hypotonic limb appears weak and floppy. There may be fasciculations.

Hypertonia The hypertonic limb appears stiff, and is often held in an extensor posture.

Associated conditions

Hypotonia Hypotonia may have its origin within the CNS, or it may be caused by a peripheral lesion (see **Table 9.3**). The assessment of hypotonia involves the whole neurological examination, looking for other, accompanying features to establish the likely cause, such as weakness or absent reflexes. If associated with weakness, the cause of the hypotonia is most likely neuromuscular.

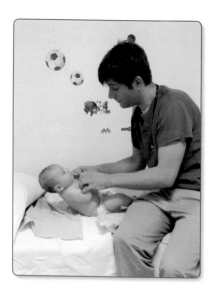

Figure 9.5 Head stays in line on 'pull to sit'.

Hypertonia Increased tone suggests a central lesion, as occurs in cerebral palsy, of which the commonest variant is spastic diplegia – a predominance of weakness and spasticity involving the lower limbs.

Power and muscle function

Definition Weakness may be caused by any abnormality along the pathway from brain to spinal cord, anterior horn cell, peripheral nerve, neuromuscular junction and muscle fibres (see **Table 9.1** and **Table 9.2**). Power is measured in older children (about 5 years of age and older) using the Medical Research Council grading system (**Table 9.8**).

Approach For infants and non-mobile children, power is inferred during the general and developmental assessment (by looking at head lag and trunk control; see Chapter 5).

Mobile children should be observed walking, cruising or crawling.

Appearance Clues to weakness in a muscle group may be apparent. Does the child prefer one hand or one side? Does the gait suggest a hemiplegia?

Observe the child getting up from the sitting position on the floor, because difficulty doing this may suggest a proximal muscle weakness.

Associated conditions A child who gets up by placing the hands on the thighs to help push up (the Gower sign) has proximal muscle weakness. This suggests a muscular dystrophy. Look at the muscles – in this condition, there may be wasting, or there may be hypertrophy of the lower limb musculature and an exaggerated lumbar lordosis.

Localised weakness and muscle wasting may be seen in peripheral nerve injuries. In Erb palsy, the arm is internally rotated and the forearm is extended and pronated (the 'waiter's tip' posture) as a result of a brachial plexus injury caused by the shoulder being trapped in the birth canal.

Co-ordination and movements

Definition Co-ordination involves the integration of moving groups of muscles, instructed by nerves, measured and fed back using sensation (joint position, vision and touch). Large areas of the brain are required to perform this difficult task – the motor cortex, the basal ganglia and the cerebellum.

Power	Grade
Normal power against resistance	5
Some movement against resistance; normal antigravity movement	4
No movement against resistance but can overcome gravity	3
Movement possible, but not against gravity	2
Visible contraction but no movement at a joint	1
No muscle contraction visible	0

Table 9.8 Medical Research Council grading of muscle power.

Disordered movements suggest basal ganglia pathology, and poor co-ordination suggests a cerebellar lesion.

Approach Observation is key to the assessment of co-ordination and movement. As well as paucity of movement in neurologically affected limbs, other movement disorders may be apparent.

In an older child it should be possible to test co-ordination formally in the upper limbs by assessing finger–nose pointing and in the lower limbs by asking the child to run the heel down the shin.

Appearance Abnormal movements are called dyskinesias:

- athetoid movements are slow, writhing movements; they suggest a basal ganglia insult, such as athetoid cerebral palsy
- choreas are involuntary jerky movements

Athetoid and choreiform movements may co-exist.

Associated conditions Dyskinesias can be acute or chronic, and they may be acquired or congenital. They may occur following severe neonatal jaundice (this is termed kernicterus), or they may occur as a part of rheumatic fever (Sydenham chorea).

Tendon reflexes

The techniques for eliciting the deep tendon reflexes in children are the same as in adults. The reflexes can usually be elicited even in a young baby with the right amount of persuasion, distraction and gentle handling and with experience and practice.

> **Clinical insight**
>
> Place the younger child on the parents' lap – this way the baby may relax sufficiently for you to test the reflexes; otherwise, the child often keeps the limbs tense. Demonstrate tapping yourself or a parent with the hammer, and turn it into a game.

Definition Causing the rapid lengthening of a muscle by tapping a tendon that is attached to that muscle initiates a reflex arc that passes from the muscle to the afferent nerve and then to the spinal cord, from where it is relayed to the efferent nerve, producing contraction of the muscle.

Testing the reflexes tests this relay circuit:
- brisk reflexes suggest a CNS problem, because the descending inhibition from the cerebral cortex to the spinal cord is diminished
- absent or reduced reflexes suggest a problem in the spinal cord, nerve or muscle

Approach As in an adult examination, ensure that the patient is correctly exposed and is relaxed. The reflex may be easier to elicit if the patient clenches the teeth just as the exposed tendon is struck with the tendon hammer.

Appearance Watch the muscle that is supposed to contract. It should quickly contract, then relax.

Associated conditions

Hyper-reflexia If the reflexes appear brisk, either in isolation or more globally, then the main consideration is in relation to developmental disorders such as spastic cerebral palsy. Therefore, you should look for other corroborating evidence to help confirm this suspicion:
- increased tone
- clonus
- weakness
- muscle wasting

Other generalised conditions may be associated with hyper-reflexia (e.g. acute disseminated encephalomyelitis, which may present with multifocal neurological symptoms and signs and which represents postviral demyelination).

Reduced reflexes or areflexia A genuine loss of reflexes or a reduced reflex requires focused investigation in order to establish the likely site of the problem (**Table 9.9**).

Sensation

There are five modalities of sensation in the limbs that can be tested:
- light touch
- sharp touch and pain
- vibration

Unilateral localised conditions	Bilateral or generalised conditions
Spinal tumour	Spinal muscular atrophy
Disc protrusion (rare in children)	Peripheral neuropathy, e.g. Guillain–Barré syndrome
Syringomyelia	
Acute myelitis	

Table 9.9 Causes of loss of a deep tendon reflex.

- joint position (proprioception)
- temperature

Testing sensory modalities gives information about the afferent nerves returning to the spinal cord from sense organs in the skin and joints, and about the routes that this information then takes in the spinal cord (the anterolateral and dorsal columns).

Approach In a child who is old enough to co-operate, the important principle when assessing sensation is to 'blind' competing sensory inputs. For example, if examining joint position sense, ask the child to close the eyes. Then, take the child's fingertip by the lateral borders and move it up and down, asking the child to say when the finger is moved and in what direction. If the examiner holds the child's fingertip with his or her fingers on top and beneath (i.e. touching the fingernail and the pulp of the finger) then when the finger is moved, light touch sensation will inform the child about what direction the finger is moving in. This means that proprioception is not being tested properly.

Test light touch using cotton wool, sharp touch with a blunt hat pin or an 'orange stick'. Test temperature using a cold spray or warm hands, and vibration with a tuning fork.

Appearance An absence of sensation should be obvious if tested for correctly. A diagram of the skin dermatomes will act as a useful aid to examining sensation.

Associated conditions Sensation is rarely affected in children unless they have a peripheral neuropathy. There are many causes of peripheral neuropathy:

- genetic, e.g. Charcot–Marie–Tooth disease
- infection, e.g. poliovirus infection, Lyme disease
- post-infectious disease, e.g. Guillain Barre syndrome
- drugs, e.g. phenytoin
- toxins, e.g. lead paint

Cerebellar examination

Definition The cerebellum is responsible for co-ordinating motor movements.

Approach and appearance Assess the gait, looking for the wide-based gait of cerebellar ataxia. Look for nystagmus, and listen for signs of dysarthria as the child talks. Observe the limb movements, and in particular the movements of the upper limbs. Assess for any evidence of intention tremor by testing hand-to-mouth movements or asking the child to hold objects. In young children it is not possible to perform more sophisticated tests of cerebellar function. In older children, the tests follow the same lines as for in an adult (**Table 9.10**).

Associated conditions Acute cerebellar signs may present following a viral infection, in particular varicella, which causes a cerebellitis (see Clinical scenario, below). This is usually a

| Dysdiadochokinesis |
| Ataxia |
| Nystagmus |
| Intention tremor |
| Slurred speech |
| Hypotonia |

Table 9.10 Signs of cerebellar disease (mnemonic: danish).

benign self-limiting condition. However, there are other causes that can have a much more serious implication, for example:

- an acute presentation of a posterior fossa tumour, which may be also associated with other neurological signs, such as a paralytic squint
- stroke, which may present with cerebellar signs
- acute drug toxicity, which is particularly likely in young children, who have accidentally taken an overdose of pills found lying around the house

Primitive and protective reflexes

Definition The primitive reflexes are reflexes that humans are born with, including:

- the Moro reflex
- the asymmetrical tonic neck reflex
- the sucking or 'rooting' reflex
- the grasp reflex
- the stepping reflex

These reflexes mimic movements that may have been important in protecting us when we were newborns during our various stages of evolution into *Homo sapiens*. They must be lost (i.e. children must 'grow out of them') before they can perform the task that they mimic (e.g. the stepping reflex must be lost before a child can begin to walk).

If the primitive reflexes persist beyond the normal age limits, or if they are very exaggerated, there may be an underlying neurological abnormality, but this is not specific to any one disorder. Persisting primitive reflexes raise concerns regarding abnormal neurological development.

The primitive reflexes have usually disappeared by 4 months of age, and if they still present at 6 months of age, then underlying serious central neurological disorder is highly likely.

Moro reflex With the infant lying prone; gently lift up the head, then allow the head to drop a short distance suddenly (**Figure 9.6**).

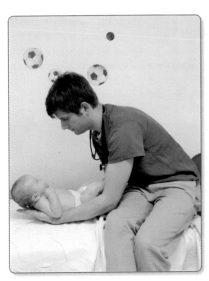

Figure 9.6 The Moro reflex is elicited by allow the head to drop back slightly.

Look for the initial symmetrical abduction of arms, often accompanied by a startled look on the baby's face, followed by arm adduction. The reflex is sometimes called the startle reflex.

In very exaggerated responses, a simple slight noise can cause the reflex. An asymmetrical response may suggest a unilateral neurological abnormality, such as a hemiplegia or Erb palsy.

Asymmetrical tonic neck reflex   The asymmetrical tonic neck reflex can often simply be observed. As infants turn the head from one side to the other, they tend to extend the arm and leg on the side to which they are turning and to flex the contralateral side. (This is often described as the fencing posture.) Normally, infants go in and out of the asymmetrical tonic neck reflex naturally as they turn from side to side, but it is abnormal if there is pervasiveness of the response, i.e. if they maintain the posture for more than a few seconds in any one direction. To demonstrate the reflex actively, put the baby on the bed in the prone position, and gently turning the head to one side by placing the palm of one hand on the side of the head. As the head turns, watch the ipsilateral arm and leg extend outwards towards the direction of the head while the contralateral limbs flexes. Normally the baby will only adopt this posture for a few seconds.

Sucking or 'rooting' reflex Stroke the side of the infant's mouth, and the infant will turn their mouth to try to suck; this is 'rooting' (see **Figure 9.7**).

Then use a finger and allow the baby to take it into the mouth; the baby will suck vigorously, at least until realising that there is no milk coming out.

Grasp reflex Stroke the palm or sole with a finger, and the baby will flex the fingers or toes to grasp your finger. If the baby is already in the flexed position, just gently stroke the dorsal aspect of the hand or foot, and they will extend; then the reflex can be demonstrated (see Chapter 3).

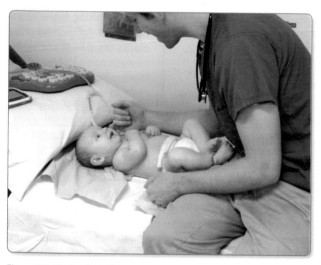

Figure 9.7 The 'rooting' reflex.

A 10-year-old boy with acute symmetrical lower limb weakness

A boy presents with a 4-day history of increasing weakness of his legs. He was playing football when the symptoms started, and he felt tired and thought he had been overdoing it. There has also been some lower back pain. His parents had thought he must have a viral illness and asked him not to play football. Now his lower legs and thighs feel weak. The pain is getting worse. There is no tingling, and he is passing urine well, although he is a bit constipated. There are no problems with his arms, and there are no headaches or fevers. He has no other symptoms, such as cough or abdominal pain.

He is normally fit and well, although about 2 weeks ago he had food poisoning, with some bloody diarrhoea, after coming back from a family holiday in Egypt. This got better with antibiotics prescribed by his GP. He is fully immunised.

Differential diagnoses

Limb weakness may have either a central or a peripheral cause (**Table 9.12**)

Further information

General assessment shows him to be alert, interacting normally, and with no obvious facial weakness. His vital signs, including temperature, are normal. He is able to walk very slowly, and he complains of weakness and pain in his lower back as he walks.

You review the arms first, and these reveal normal power, tone and tendon reflexes. Neurological examination of the upper limbs is normal.

Examination of the legs shows no evidence of muscle wasting or fasciculation, and there is no tenderness on palpation of the muscles. There is significant weakness and reduced muscle tone of all muscle groups, including the muscles of ankle dorsiflexion, plantar flexion and knee and hip extension and flexion. His knee and ankle reflexes are reduced. Sensation seems normal.

Examination of the lower back reveals no overlying swelling and no localised tenderness, and there is full range of movements.

Central causes	Peripheral causes
Acute Encephalitis	Acute myelitis
Acute disseminated encephalomyelitis	Anterior horn cell infection
	Peripheral neuropathy, e.g. Guillain–Barré syndrome
	Botulism
	Acute myasthenia gravis
	Acute myositis

Table 9.12 Key central and peripheral causes of limb weakness.

Concluding differential diagnosis

There is clinical evidence of an acute flaccid paralysis of both lower limbs. There are no CNS signs or symptoms, so it appears to be a peripheral problem. The location of the problem could be anywhere from the spinal cord out to the muscle. An acute transverse myelitis could be present and will need to be excluded, but there is no sphincter disturbance so this is less likely.

An infection of the anterior horn cell such as poliomyelitis is unlikely because the features are very symmetrical and he is fully immunised. There is no tenderness of the muscle, so an acute myositis is unlikely and would in any case not explain the flaccid paralysis. There is no history to support botulism, a very rare disease. Acute myasthenia is rare, and there is no facial or upper limb abnormality in this case.

Guillain–Barré syndrome is the commonest cause of acute flaccid paralysis and is the most likely cause in this case. In children with Guillain–Barré syndrome, there is often a motor effect only, with sensation preserved, as with this boy. There is a strong association with

Clinical insight

Key points from this chapter:

- identify the problem – weakness, hypotonia, spasticity or ataxia
- examine to identify the site of the lesion – CNS, peripheral nerve, neuromuscular junction or muscle fibre
- use the history to identify the cause

recent *Campylobacter* infection, which was a likely cause of the bloody diarrhoea in this case.

The other main differential diagnosis is transverse myelitis, and an MRI of the spine is indicated, followed (if the MRI is normal) by a lumbar puncture looking for the raised CSF protein of Guillain–Barré syndrome, together with nerve conduction studies to confirm the diagnosis.

Bones, joints and muscles

The scope of musculoskeletal disorders in children is wide and quite distinct from that in adults. This chapter describes some of the musculoskeletal disorders that affect children and the approach to clinical examination.

10.1 Common presentations

Key musculoskeletal presentations in children include:
- acute limp
- single joint swelling
- polyarthritis

Acute limp

Limp can be caused by musculoskeletal or neurological problems; this chapter concentrates on the former. Trauma is a common cause of limp, including what is called a toddler fracture. A toddler fracture is a spiral fracture, usually of the distal tibia, that is caused by a simple twisting injury; it often goes unnoticed. It is imperative that trauma and any resultant injury are excluded as the cause of an acute limp.

The other common, non-traumatic musculoskeletal causes of limp are inflammation or infection of the bone or joints. Rarely, a malignancy, such as a bone tumour or acute leukaemia, presents with a limp.

Four conditions that cause an acute limp in toddlers and younger children are:
- transient synovitis, most commonly seen in 3–10 year olds
- septic arthritis
- osteomyelitis
- Perthes disease (avascular necrosis of the femoral head), most commonly seen in 6–12 year olds
- slipped upper femoral epiphysis (SUFE), most commonly seen in 10–17 year olds

Transient synovitis

Transient synovitis (also known as 'irritable hip') is a common condition that affects the hip in toddlers and younger children.

It can present in a similar way to septic arthritis, and it is important to differentiate clinically between the two conditions.

Pathology The most likely cause is a synovitis that is a reactive response to a recent viral infection, often an upper respiratory tract infection. Although transient synovitis may result in a joint effusion, the condition is harmless, and any fluid aspirated from the effusion will be sterile.

Clinical features In contrast to a child with septic arthritis, children with transient synovitis are systemically well and may be afebrile. There is normally a history of preceding viral infection. The child may hold the hip in a flexed position at rest and may resist passive movement of the affected hip.

Septic arthritis

Septic arthritis is a condition that must not be missed, because delay in treatment can result in permanent damage to the joint.

Pathology Septic arthritis is caused by a bacterial infection of the joint capsule. The most common causative organisms are *Staphylococcus aureus* and *Streptococcus pyogenes*. In most cases, bacteria have reached the joint via haematogenous spread or via direct spread from an adjacent osteomyelitis. Septic arthritis may also occur after trauma or after iatrogenic procedures, e.g. joint aspiration.

Clinical features Important signs and symptoms of septic arthritis are:
- joint pain (arthralgia) on active and passive movement
- restriction of joint movement as a result of the pain
- fever and systemic upset
- joint swelling, warmth and erythema (though these may be difficult to assess in the hip)

Osteomyelitis

Osteomyelitis is another important condition not to miss, because chronic osteomyelitis can affect bone growth (**Figure 10.1**). It is most commonly seen in infants and toddlers and becomes less common as children get older.

Pathology Osteomyelitis is an infection of bone that most commonly occurs in the metaphysis of bones such as the femur or tibia. The causative organisms are similar to those for septic arthritis, *S. aureus* being the commonest. Osteomyelitis is commoner in children with sickle cell disease, and in these children it may be caused by *Salmonella* spp. Most cases of osteomyelitis develop through haematogenous spread of the infecting organism.

Clinical features Infants and toddlers with osteomyelitis may present with:
- non-specific symptoms of feeling or seeming unwell
- poor feeding
- fever, which is often low-grade
- restriction of movement in the affected limb
- crying and discomfort when the limb is passively moved

Perthes disease

Perthes disease is an avascular necrosis of the femoral head that affects boys more often than girls.

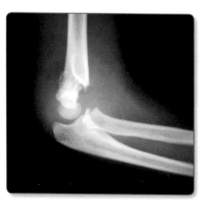

Figure 10.1 Chronic osteomyelitis in the elbow, which has affected bone growth.

Pathology Perthes disease is characterised by an idiopathic avascular necrosis of the femoral head (**Figure 10.2**). This causes deformity and flattening of the head of the femur, which can lead to osteoarthritis in later life.

Clinical features Perthes disease can present over the course of weeks, with the child complaining of increasing pain in the hip. The pain is described as an ache, which causes the child to restrict movement and to limp in order to minimise weight-bearing on the affected side. The condition may also present with referred pain to the knee.

On examination there may be an antalgic gait and restricted movement in the affected hip joint.

Slipped upper femoral epiphysis
SUFE classically affects overweight teenagers; it is more common in males.

Pathology In SUFE, there is movement (slippage) through the growth plate of the proximal femur, so that the epiphysis stays in the acetabulum and the proximal femoral metaphysis moves superiorly and anteriorly (**Figure 10.3**).

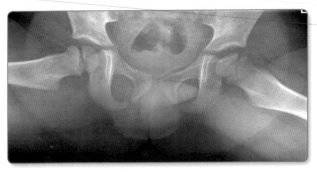

Figure 10.2 Perthes disease (avascular necrosis of the femoral head). Note the normal growth plate at the head of the right femur, and the abnormal appearance at the head of the left femur.

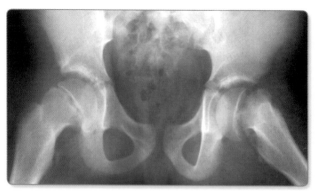

Figure 10.3 Left-sided slipped upper femoral epiphysis (SUFE).

Clinical features Symptoms and signs of SUFE are:
- pain in the hip or knee
- antalgic or waddling gait
- discrepancy in leg length, with the affected leg being shorter
- a hip joint that is held in external rotation

Single joint swelling
Swelling in a single joint has a wide range of possible causes, including trauma and septic arthritis (see above). Other important conditions that can cause single joint swelling are:
- reactive arthritis
- haemarthrosis

Reactive arthritis
Reactive arthritis is a form of arthritis that can occur after common viral and bacterial infections.

Pathology The arthritis itself is sterile and no organisms are seen in joint fluid aspiration, even though the arthritis is associated with infection somewhere else in the body. Reactive arthritis is thought to be due to an autoimmune process whereby molecular mimicry results in joint inflammation. (The immune system initiates a reaction to the synovial tissue, mistaking it for foreign antigen.)

Clinical features Reactive arthritis presents with features similar to those of septic arthritis, and the two conditions are often confused. The main features are:
- a history of preceding infection (often gastrointestinal)
- joint swelling and effusion
- arthralgia
- restriction of movement

Haemarthrosis

Haemarthrosis is bleeding into a joint capsule. It often affects the knee joint.

Pathology In children, the two main causes of haemarthrosis are X-linked haemophilia and trauma. Haemophilia is the most likely diagnosis when there is no history of trauma, but even with evidence of trauma it must be considered. A significant traumatic haemarthrosis often results from a ligamentous tear (e.g. of the anterior cruciate ligament).

Clinical features There is often a history of trauma, but haemarthrosis can occur spontaneously. The main feature is swelling of the joint. There may also be bruising around the joint. The child is often in pain, and there is restricted joint movement.

Polyarthritis

Polyarthritis is relatively uncommon in childhood. There are a wide variety of rare causes; two important causes are:
- juvenile idiopathic arthritis (JIA)
- rheumatic Fever

Juvenile idiopathic arthritis

JIA is the commonest cause of polyarthritis in childhood. It can present in a variety of ways depending on the subtype. The main subtypes are:
- systemic-onset JIA
- persistent or extended oligoarthritis
- rheumatoid factor-positive polyarthritis
- rheumatoid factor-negative polyarthritis
- psoriatic JIA

- enthesitis-related arthritis
- undifferentiated JIA

Pathology The pathogenesis of JIA is still not completely understood. There is thought to be an autoimmune component, with complex genetics playing a role, particularly in certain subsets. Environmental factors are also believed to be involved (e.g. possible viral triggers in predisposed children).

Clinical features The presentation of JIA depends on the subset, but generally it involves joint pain and swelling, with some restriction of function.

The joint symptoms are typically worse in the morning and ease as the day progresses. The number of joints that are involved depends on the subset, with oligoarthritis generally involving four joints or fewer, whereas polyarthritis involves multiple joints.

In addition to joint involvement, a child with systemic-onset JIA will also present with fevers, a pale pink rash and lethargy.

The diagnosis of JIA is usually made once symptoms have been present for 6 weeks or more.

Rheumatic fever

Rheumatic fever is now an uncommon disease in developed countries but it is still seen across the world in developing countries.

Pathology Rheumatic fever is an autoimmune disorder that occurs as a complication of infection with *S. pyogenes* (often as part of tonsillitis). The immune reaction can affect a number of tissues. In particular, it can affect the heart, causing carditis in the acute phase; this can lead later to fibrosis and valve disease, particularly mitral stenosis.

Clinical features Rheumatic fever is diagnosed using the Duckett–Jones criteria (**Table 10.1**). The diagnosis is made if there is evidence of recent infection with *S. pyogenes* together with either two major criteria, or one major criterion and two minor criteria.

Major criteria
Carditis
Polyarthritis (migrating)
Erythema marginatum
Subcutaneous nodules
Sydenham's chorea
Minor criteria
Previous history of rheumatic fever
Fever
Arthralgia
PR interval prolongation on ECG
Raised ESR or C-reactive protein
Raised leukocyte count

Table 10.1 The Duckett–Jones criteria for the diagnosis of rheumatic fever.

10.2 Musculoskeletal examination

The musculoskeletal examination needs to be adapted to the presenting problem. Some children present with generalised joint symptoms and may require a full examination of all joints. Others will require focused examination of a specific joint, in addition to a general assessment and possibly a paediatric 'gait, arms, legs and spine' examination (a pGALS screen). Additionally specific approaches to the examination are needed when there has been traumatic injury and when there has been suspected child maltreatment.

A sequence for examining musculoskeletal function is:
- general inspection
- 'look, feel, move'
- pGALS examination
- focused assessment of specific joints
- assessment of trauma
- assessment for child maltreatment

General inspection

As with all assessments, the first thing to do is to stand back and watch. If a child is suffering from a painful condition, the examiner who causes discomfort may lose the opportunity to gain useful information from the assessment.

Even before any focused assessment, there may be important clues in general:

- gait, which can give an indication of the functional effect of any disorders
- growth and nutritional state – children with chronic musculoskeletal problems often have poor growth
- joint deformity – some joint problems will be obvious even from a distance
- rashes – skin disease is linked to many musculoskeletal problems
- clues around the bed (e.g. splints, crutches)
- ethnicity – children with darker skin have a greater risk of developing rickets

'Look, feel, move'

The 'look, feel, move' approach is a logical and systematic way of ensuring that all the important clues are detected. In a compliant school-age child, pGALS (a supplementary tool that is a paediatric version of the adult GALS) has been devised, to ensure that all main joints are assessed, mostly through an approach using active commands.

Look

Start by looking at the following:

- posture
- guarding
- deformity
- swelling
- erythema
- bruising
- active movement

Posture The posture of the child offers clues to the problem; for example:

- a child who has an acute scoliosis may have some inflammatory intra-abdominal lesion
- a child who is holding the arm extended, parallel to the body and internally rotated is exhibiting the classic sign of a 'pulled' elbow

Guarding A child who is holding the hand over an affected area, such as one hand being held over the other wrist, is exhibiting powerful evidence to suggest a significant injury of the protected area.

Deformity Any clinically apparent deformity can give a clue to an underlying fracture or other pathology.

Muscle wasting is an important sign (atrophy suggests prolonged under-use, possibly due to pain) and muscles surrounding affected joints should be assessed.

Swelling As with deformity, swelling directs attention to an underlying disease process such as effusion in a joint swelling, a fracture or a bone tumour. However, this sign can be subtle and needs focus and an index of suspicion to ensure that it is not missed. A careful comparison with the unaffected side is needed. Some areas (such as the hip joint) are not easily assessed for swelling.

Erythema Erythema should be noted, although this sign is non-specific. It may represent a number of possible conditions (**Table 10.2**), including infection, injury and inflammation.

Bruising Bruising is simply a signpost to possible underlying injury. A bruise goes through a number of colour changes but the timing of these changes is highly variable, and not all the stages may occur. There is no evidence to support any attempt to estimate the timing of an injury on the basis of the colour of the bruise, and incorrect assertions on this point have led to difficulty during expert evidence in child protection investigations.

Cellulitis
Early stages of bruising
Septic arthritis
Osteomyelitis
inflammatory arthritis

Table 10.2 Causes of erythema over a bone or joint.

Active movement Ask the child to move the affected area. For example, if the child is complaining of a painful wrist, ask for the wrist to be flexed and extended in order to assess the range of movements. See the section on pGALS (below) for an easily used tool for screening for joint problems in school-age children.

Feel

Palpate the area in question (or all the joints) and assess for:

- tenderness
- temperature
- crepitus
- fluid thrill

Tenderness Gently palpate the affected area. Observe the child's face for grimacing or signs of pain. Be aware that some children complain of pain with the slightest touch whereas others are more stoical and can tolerate more pain before they react. This can make assessment difficult, and may lead to both over- and under-diagnosis of significant pathology.

Palpation should follow an orderly sequence, ensuring that the whole area of concern is examined adequately and that any localised or point tenderness is not missed. The whole joint margin should be palpated whenever possible. (Some deep joints, such as the hip, are not amenable to full palpation.) The relevant muscle and bone should be examined carefully.

Temperature Feel the joint with the back of a hand, and compare the temperature with that of the other side. An increased temperature suggests an infection or an inflammatory joint disorder.

Crepitus Gently flex and extend a joint. Crepitus is felt as a 'creaking' or 'bubbling'. Its presence suggests an inflammatory or degenerative change within the joint.

Fluid thrill Examining for a fluid thrill is particular for the knees, and if present it is a sign of an effusion.

A 'patellar tap' test is performed to assess for fluid in the knee:
1. Place a hand over the leg above the patella and move it down to just above the upper border of the patella, squeezing out any fluid in the suprapatellar pouch
2. With the index finger of the other hand, press over the patella
3. Palpate and observe for a 'bouncing' movement of the patella off the femur. This is a patellar tap. Its presence suggests increased fluid in the joint space

Move

If the child is compliant, ask him or her to move joints in all directions (as relevant to that joint). In a younger child, it is possible to infer the integrity of joint function by observation of the child's movements and actions. Before passively performing joint range of movements, look and feel for any resistance or pain, and note any restriction of movement.

In the older age group – once a child is old enough to follow commands –the pGALS approach can be used.

Paediatric 'gait, arms, legs and spine' examination

The pGALS is a modified paediatric version of the GALS approach to examine the gait, arms, legs and spine. It is a useful way to approach the musculoskeletal examination, and it covers the majority of likely problems. However, it is suitable for use only in an older, compliant, school-age child. Videos of it being used are available on the internet.

In the outline of pGALS below, there are some direct instructions to the examiner, and the rest of the commands are for the patient (shown in 'inverted commas').

Gait

The pGALS examination of the gait:
1. Observe the patient walking
2. 'Walk on your heels'
3. 'Walk on your tip-toes'

Arms

The pGALS examination of the arms:
1. 'Put your hands out in front of you'
2. 'Turn your hand over and make a fist'
3. 'Touch the tips of your fingers'
4. Squeeze the metacarpophalangeal joints
5. 'Put your hands and wrists together'
6. 'Put your hands back to back'
7. 'Reach up as far as you can'
8. 'Look at the ceiling'
9. 'Put your hands behind your neck'

Legs

The pGALS examination of the legs:
1. Feel for effusion at the knee
2. 'Bring your ankle up to your bottom'
3. Assess passive movement of hip and knee, including rotation of the hip

Spine

The pGALS examination of the spine:
1. 'Place your ear on your shoulder'
2. 'Open your mouth wide and place 3 fingers inside'
3. Observe the curvature of the spine from the side and from behind
4. 'Bend forwards.

Focused assessment of specific joints

When a child presents with pathology in one joint, it is important to assess this joint in detail, as well as screening the whole musculoskeletal system. This section contains some important information about the spine, hips and knees.

Spine

The spine should be assessed in its entirety. After the general assessment, assess each region of the spine from the neck downwards.

General assessment Look for any spinal deformity. With the full spine exposed, look at the spine from the cervical spine all the way down to the coccyx. As well as the child's posture, note any 'steps' in the spine and any overlying swelling or redness, and palpate for any areas of tenderness.

An area of tenderness may suggest

- an underlying fracture (if there is history of trauma)
- a muscular strain
- an alignment abnormality (e.g. spondylolisthesis)
- an infection (e.g. spinal tuberculosis, discitis)

Cervical spine Check for the neck posture – a cervical spine lesion may give rise to some form of head tilt, such as torticollis. In this scenario always consider an intracranial lesion, which may in fact be the ultimate cause of any apparent cervical spine abnormality, with the head tilt being a compensation for an acute squint.

Look at the size of the neck and assess whether it appears short. A short neck can occur in certain syndromes (such as Turner syndrome; see Chapter 15), and also in conditions such as Klippel–Feil disease, in which there is fusion of two or more of the cervical vertebrae.

Assess movement; in younger children this can be done by observation and using distraction techniques to get the child to rotate the neck to the left and right and up and down, as far as possible. Gently attempt to assess passive movement, although the child may well resist this. It can be difficult in young children to know whether this resistance is due to a lack of co-operation or to a genuinely painful abnormality.

Thoracic spine Review posture, in particular looking for any evidence of a scoliosis (**Table 10.3**) or a kyphosis, or both. Observe flexion and extension and lateral movement of the spine, looking for any restriction of movement.

| Idiopathic (80% of cases) |
| Congenital |
| Associated with a neurological disorder, e.g. cerebral palsy, muscular dystrophy |
| Secondary to intra-abdominal inflammation, e.g. appendix abscess |
| Spinal tumour |

Table 10.3 Causes of scoliosis.

Lumbosacral spine Review the normal lordosis. It may be exaggerated in conditions such as muscular dystrophy, and it may be reduced in inflammatory diseases of the lumbar spine. Observe forward flexion and extension.

The sacroiliac joints can be examined by taking hold of the outer aspects of the pelvis and pressing inwards, to identify the pain of sacroiliitis.

Hip

Approach In an ambulant child, examination of the hips starts with observing the gait, because disorders of the hip may present with an antalgic gait.

The rest of the examination follows the 'look, feel, move' format. As well as looking at the child's gait, you should look for any obvious deformity of the joint.

There is little to feel on the surface because the hip joint is deep, but you should assess the six key movements of the hip, both actively and passively:
- flexion–extension
- internal rotation–external rotation
- adduction–abduction

Appearance A child with an antalgic gait leans to the side of the painful hip and takes a rapid, quite heavy step, followed by a slower step on the unaffected side. In the younger child who is not yet walking, there may be reduced movements on the side that is affected by pathology, or there may be noticeable flexion and external rotation of the hip when the child is placed in the supine position. When lifted up to stand, the child may again keep the hip flexed, with reluctance to bear weight on the affected side.

Associated conditions The abnormalities of hip position and movement described above are non-specific signs. They generally indicate that the child has hip pain, but any pathology of the upper leg (e.g. a femoral fracture, osteomyelitis, slipped upper femoral epiphysis) may present in these ways.

There are a number of very important causes of hip pain in children, and the age of the child is important when assessing the likely cause (**Table 10.4**). Clearly any list of likely causes as determined by age is only a guide, and overlap occurs (e.g. infection of bone and joints can occur in all ages, but it occurs most commonly in infants and young children).

Knee

Approach As with all lower limb examinations, start with an assessment of the gait if the child is ambulant. Then follow the 'look, feel, move' examination format. Fully expose the joint and look at its position and characteristics:

- feel the knee for tenderness – assess all regions of the joint, including the medial and lateral collateral ligaments, the joint line, the tibial tuberosity and the patella

0–3 years of age	3–10 years of age	> 10 years of age
Developmental dysplasia	Perthes (avascular necrosis of the femoral head) (see **Figure 10.2**)	SUFE (see **Figure 10.3**)
Septic arthritis	Transient synovitis (irritable hip)	Reactive arthritis
Osteomyelitis		Avulsion fractures, e.g. anterior superior iliac spine fracture
SUFE, slipped upper femoral capital epiphysis.		

Table 10.4 Guide to the commonest causes of hip pain in children at different ages.

- try to elicit a patellar tap if there is an effusion in the knee joint – milk the fluid down from the suprapatellar pouch and look for filling around the knee, and then push the patella down and try to feel a tap as it hits the femur
- move the knee joint, both actively and passively, if the child allows; flexion and extension are the main movements of the knee, but also apply varus and valgus stresses with the knee straight, to detect collateral ligament strain or instability
- assess the cruciate ligaments in the same way as for adults, using the 'draw' and 'sag' tests

Appearance The knee position may be abnormal if there is pathology; in particular, the knee may be held in partial flexion. If this is the case, estimate the degree of flexion.

The knee may appear internally rotated; this occurs in femoral anteversion, which is a common, self-limiting condition that is seen in young children.

Note whether there is any evidence of erythema or swelling in the joint. Look at the quadriceps muscle for signs of atrophy.

Associated conditions The knee may be held in flexion when there has been acute trauma to the knee or in chronic arthritis. Other positional variants are genu valgum ('knock-knees', which can cause persisting knee pain) and genu varum. Both of these positions can be normal variants in children of certain ages, but they may also be a sign of knee pathology.

Erythema, swelling and tenderness of the knee joints can all be signs of inflammation or infection. Always consider septic arthritis in children who present with an acute knee problem. JIA may also present in a similar way, but there may be other joints affected or atrophy of the surrounding muscles. Isolated swelling of the knee joint may also be due to a haemarthrosis, which can occur in X-linked haemophilia.

Restriction of knee movement may be due to acute pathology (e.g. trauma, septic arthritis, osteomyelitis) or to chronic pathology (e.g. JIA). In both cases, the movement is restricted either by pain or (less commonly) by damage to the knee structures (e.g. a ligamentous tear, a fracture).

Trauma

The majority of children who require a musculoskeletal assessment will have a history of some form of trauma or a history suggestive of an injury. An example of the latter might be a toddler who has suddenly stopping walking. One of the likeliest scenarios in this case is that the toddler has sustained a small spiral or oblique fracture to the distal tibia or fibula (the so-called toddler fracture) as a result of a simple twisting movement, without any direct trauma observed by the carers.

Examination in the trauma setting

The assessment of a suspected limb fracture follows the general assessment outlined above – 'look, feel, move'. In a setting of major trauma, always approach the child in an 'ABC' format – assessing the airway, breathing and circulation – as part of the primary survey before moving on to assess specific joints in the secondary survey.

The most important features include the presence of:

- a clinical deformity (**Figure 10.4**)
- an overlying skin breach

Deformity means not only that some form of manipulative treatment is needed, but it also raises the possibility that

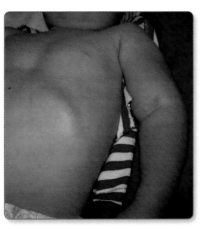

Figure 10.4 Deformity of the left arm, with bruising.

there may be some neurovascular compromise. The pulses distal to the deformity must be checked, and sensation assessed.

An open fracture is said to have occurred when there is any skin breach over a fracture site. A child with an open fracture should be given immediate intravenous antibiotics, and early surgery is required. There is a significant risk of osteomyelitis.

Assessment of a fracture

The presence of the growth plate in children's bones makes the diagnosis and assessment of fractures much more complicated than it is in adults. Even if an X-ray is normal, a fracture may be present. The fracture may occur through the non-ossified area – a Salter–Harris type 1 fracture (**Figure 10.5**). Therefore, the key to diagnosis is in the clinical findings. If there is localised tenderness over a growth plate on clinical examination, then a fracture is likely and the injury should be managed as such, even if the X-ray is normal.

Supracondylar fracture One of the commonest fractures posing a risk of neurovascular compromise in children is the supracondylar fracture – a fracture above the elbow joint) (**Figures 10.6** and **10.7**). If the fracture causes dorsal displacement of the distal fragment of the bone, then the anterior proximal fragment can impinge on the brachial artery. It is crucial

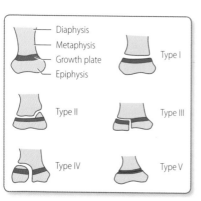

Figure 10.5 Salter–Harris classification of fractures. The type V Salter–Harris fracture is a compression of the growth plate.

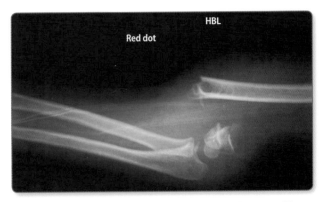

Figure 10.6 Severely displaced supracondylar fracture. This fracture would raise immediate concerns about the risk of neurovascular impairment.

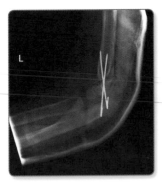

Figure 10.7 A repaired supracondylar fracture with K wires inserted.

that the radial pulse should be palpated immediately and that the perfusion of the hand should be checked. If there is any suggestion that the arterial supply has been compromised, then immediate manipulation of the elbow is undertaken – this is usually done in the emergency department, under opiate analgesia.

Child maltreatment

Children who have been maltreated may present with symptoms or signs involving the skeleton in the absence of any history of trauma. However, there are some situations in which it is known that injury can occur even in the absence of a clear history of trauma – traumatic events that are so trivial that they go unnoticed, such as a spiral fracture of the tibia caused by a very minor twisting movement in a young child (a 'toddler fracture').

Do not assume

It is very important, when faced with an unexplained injury, that you assess each case carefully and non-judgementally. Clearly if a significant injury is present but no mechanism of trauma is offered, a full investigation into the possibility of child maltreatment must be undertaken. No injury can tell us for sure that a child has been abused, but some injuries are more likely than not to have been inflicted (e.g. a long bone fracture in a non-ambulant child).

Look further

When it is thought that a fracture may have been inflicted, a careful assessment of the whole skeleton is undertaken, both through clinical examination and by a full radiographic survey (a skeletal survey). This examination and survey can detect old and current fractures; the presence of multiple fractures of varying ages is highly suspicious.

As well as looking for fractures, the child should be carefully examined for bruises, and younger children should be examined for retinal haemorrhages.

Detailed discussion on all aspects of child maltreatment is outside the scope of this book. What is absolutely crucial for trainees when faced with a child who may have been abused is to inform a senior member of the medical staff immediately. Do not in any circumstances inform the parents of any suspicions. Document in the notes exactly why suspicions arose.

> ## Clinical insight
>
> If you are suspicious about child maltreatment during an assessment, immediately inform senior staff, document the concerns, and do not tell the parents.

10.3 Clinical scenarios

The four clinical scenarios below explore some of the concepts discussed in this chapter.

A 17-month-old girl who is not using her left arm

A 17-month-old toddler is brought in to the emergency department because her parents have noticed that she has not been using her left arm since she woke up. She is holding the arm extended and close to her body. They cannot recall any injury. She was with the nanny the day before. They have called the nanny, and she denies any injury, but she does recall an episode when the child refused to get up from the floor in the supermarket; when she pulled the girl up firmly by the hand, she started to cry.

Differential diagnosis

The following diagnoses should be considered:
- a fracture of the humerus, elbow or forearm
- a pulled (subluxed) elbow

Further information

The girl is holding the arm extended and adducted, but she seems in no distress. Inspection of the limb shows no swelling or redness. There is no tenderness of any part of the limb. Flexion of the elbow is resisted.

Concluding differential diagnosis

In the absence of any clear trauma other than the pulling injury, and the lack of any clinical abnormalities of swelling or tenderness, you decide to attempt a simple relocation of the radial head, treating this as a pulled or subluxed elbow. You press your thumb over the radial head, whilst flexing the girl's arm to the maximum allowed in the prone position, and then supinate the forearm at the point of maximum flexion and extend it. At that moment a 'clunk' is heard, and shortly afterwards, the patient is moving her arm normally.

A 30-month-old boy with acute limp

A 30-month-old toddler woke up with a left sided limp and is very reluctant to bear weight on that side. He is complaining of (poorly localised) pain on that side. There is no history of trauma. He has been well recently, other than having a mild cough and cold. There is no history of fevers or systemic upset. He is happy apart from the pain when walking.

Differential diagnosis
The following possibilities should be considered:
- irritable hip (transient synovitis)
- septic arthritis
- fracture

Further information
The patient looks well, happy and alert. He is lying on the couch with his left leg semiflexed and externally rotated. He has no fever or rash. There is no redness or swelling of the leg, and palpation reveals no areas of tenderness or increased warmth. Passive examination of the hip reveals slightly reduced flexion, normal external rotation, abduction and adduction, but significantly reduced internal rotation, which induces a lot of pain.

Concluding differential diagnosis
The most likely diagnosis is an irritable hip, although a septic arthritis is also possible; however, the lack of fever or systemic upset would go against this latter diagnosis. The lack of trauma makes a fracture unlikely.

An 18-month-old girl with a hot, painful ankle

An 18-month-old girl has had a swollen right ankle for the past 4 days. The ankle has become increasingly warm and tender, and she refuses to bear weight on the affected side. There was a minor injury 10 days ago when she tripped over a toy on the floor, and she has also had a bad bout of gastroenteritis, which settled 5 days ago. However, she is now having fevers up to 39°C and is off her food.

Differential diagnosis

Key differentials to consider include:
- septic arthritis
- reactive arthritis
- osteomyelitis
- fracture

Further information

The toddler appears unwell, irritable and miserable. The right ankle is swollen and tender to palpation. It is warm and there is overlying erythema. There is reduced movement of the ankle.

Concluding differential diagnosis

Septic arthritis is the main differential diagnosis to be excluded. An ultrasound scan should be done to look for a joint effusion, followed by formal exploration under general anaesthetic, with blood taken for blood cultures.

Other diagnoses are possible, but septic arthritis can quickly cause permanent joint damage so it must be diagnosed and treated promptly.

A 5-year-old boy with swollen knees and ankles

A 5-year-old boy has a 6-week history of swollen knees and ankles, which started without fevers or recent infection. There is associated pain and stiffness with reduced mobility. These symptoms are worst first thing in the morning. He is relying on regular anti-inflammatory agents to be able to walk around. He has no rash and no bowel symptoms, and he is otherwise well. Before this presenting condition there have been no medical problems. His mother has hypothyroidism.

Differential diagnosis

The history is highly suggestive of JIA, with the only other key differential being a prolonged postviral reactive arthropathy.

Further information

The boy looks well and has no fever, no rash and no hepato-splenomegaly. There is clear swelling of both knees and ankles, but all other joints appear normal, with full range of function. However, both knees and ankles reveal globally reduced range of movement in all directions. Blood tests show a raised ESR and a negative rheumatoid factor.

Concluding differential diagnosis

Systemic-onset JIA is unlikely given the lack of features such as fever, rash and hepatosplenomegaly. The rheumatoid factor is negative and hence this is not a rheumatoid factor-positive polyarthritis. The most likely differential diagnosis lies between persistent or extended oligoarthritis and rheumatoid factor-negative polyarthritis.

> ### Clinical insight
>
> Key points from this chapter:
>
> - children's bones and joints are different from those of adults
> - pain may often not be felt at all, or it may be felt away from the true problem
> - pain or impairment of function of a limb or joint must always be taken very seriously

Lumps and bumps

'Lumps and bumps' are common presenting problems in paediatrics, both in general practice and in the emergency department. Many lumps can be diagnosed clinically on the basis of the history and examination findings.

11.1 Common presentations

Key presentations of lumps and bumps include:
- lymphadenopathy
- a lump in the neck
- a lump in the groin

Lymphadenopathy

Lymph nodes are found all over the body, but they are clustered in five important sites:
- the neck
- the axilla
- the hilum of the lung
- the terminal ileum
- the groin

The commonest causes of lymph node enlargement are:
- infection
- malignancy
- autoimmune disease

Two important questions need to be considered when assessing a patient with lymphadenopathy, because the answers to these questions influence the differential diagnosis (**Table 11.1**):
1. is the lymphadenopathy acute or chronic?
2. is the lymphadenopathy local or systemic?

Infectious lymphadenopathy

Infectious lymphadenopathy is the commonest cause of lymph node enlargement in children, and one of the commonest causes of lumps in the neck overall.

Acute local lymphadenopathy	Reactive to local infection, e.g. cervical nodes in throat infection Lymphadenitis (a bacterial infection of the lymph node)
Acute systemic lymphadenopathy	Influenza Toxoplasmosis
Chronic local lymphadenopathy	*Mycobacterium avium intracellulare* (MAI) infection Lymphoma
Chronic systemic lymphadenopathy	Epstein–Barr virus HIV Systemic lupus erythematosus Leukaemia Lymphoma

Table 11.1 Some common causes of lymphadenopathy.

Pathology Viral and bacterial infections are the commonest causes of infectious lymphadenopathy. When lymphadenopathy occurs in the context of a reaction to a local infection, the affected nodes are referred to as reactive.

A lymph node may also be infected itself – lymphadenitis. The cause is usual bacterial.

Systemic infection, e.g. influenza, can also cause widespread lymphadenopathy.

Clinical features Reactive lymphadenopathy is most commonly acute (of less than 2 weeks' duration) and associated with the symptoms of an infection, e.g. a sore throat in a patient with neck lumps. The affected nodes themselves are often tender and mobile, and there may be an overlying erythema (**Figure 11.1**).

Certain infections (e.g. Epstein–Barr virus infection, HIV infection, mycobacterial infection) can also cause chronic lymphadenopathy (of more than 2 weeks' duration).

Lymphadenitis may result in a localised abscess, which may need incision and drainage.

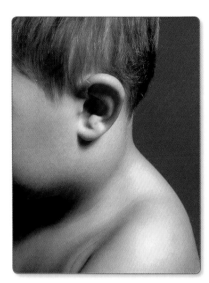

Figure 11.1 Acutely enlarged left-sided cervical lymph node.

Malignant lymphadenopathy

Malignancy is uncommon in childhood, but haematological malignancies make up a higher proportion of cancer in children than they do in adults. Malignancy (especially lymphoma) must therefore be considered in cases of lymphadenopathy.

Pathology The most common malignancies to cause lymphadenopathy are leukaemia and lymphoma. These are also some of the commonest malignancies affecting children. Because epithelial malignancies are rare in children, it is unusual to see localised lymphadenopathy caused by malignancy in children.

Clinical features Malignant lymphadenopathy is normally chronic (of more than 2 weeks' duration), but it can present in the early phase. The lymphadenopathy can be either systemic or localised; children with lymphoma classically have localised neck lymphadenopathy.

The lymphadenopathy itself is described as a group of fixed, matted nodes, which are painless and feel firm and rubbery on palpation. There may also be systemic features of the malignancy, such as anaemia, bruising, weight loss and night sweats.

Lymphadenopathy due to autoimmune disease
This is an uncommon cause of lymphadenopathy.

Pathology Various autoimmune diseases can cause lymphadenopathy, including:
- systemic lupus erythematosus
- juvenile idiopathic arthritis

Clinical features Lymphadenopathy associated with autoimmune disease is usually chronic and in most cases it is systemic. It is important that evidence of hepatosplenomegaly should be sought.

Lumps in the neck
When a patient presents with a neck lump it is important to determine which anatomical triangle the lump is in (**Table 11.2**). The most common cause of neck lumps in children is lymphadenopathy. Other important causes include:
- thyroid disease
- a tumour of the sternocleidomastoid muscle

Thyroid disease
The thyroid gland is situated in the anterior triangles of the neck. It sits in front of and to either side of the trachea and inferior to the cricoid cartilage. The thyroid can be diffusely enlarged, or there may be a nodule within the thyroid.

Pathology A wide variety of different pathologies can affect the thyroid gland, including infective, neoplastic and autoimmune processes. The most common cause of diffuse thyroid enlargement in children is autoimmune disease, caused by Graves disease, which often results in hyperthyroidism.

Clinical features A thyroid nodule may be felt within the thyroid, or the thyroid gland may be diffusely enlarged. The key feature is a midline swelling that moves with swallowing.

Anterior triangle of the neck	Posterior triangle of the neck
Anterior cervical lymphadenopathy	Posterior cervical lymphadenopathy
Submandibular lymphadenopathy	Sternocleidomastoid tumour
Submandibular gland or cyst	Cystic hygroma
Thyroid cyst, thyroid mass or diffuse enlargement of the thyroid gland	Skin or subcutaneous tissue lump (e.g. lipoma, sebaceous cyst)
Thyroglossal cyst	
Parathyroid cyst or mass	
Skin or subcutaneous tissue lump (e.g. lipoma, sebaceous cyst)	

Table 11.2 Differential diagnosis for a neck lump, based on anatomical location.

Signs and symptoms of thyroid disease (either hyperthyroidism or hypothyroidism) may also be detected and can indicate the functional effect of any thyroid enlargement.

Clinical features of thyroid disease are listed in **Table 11.3**.

Tumour of the sternocleidomastoid muscle

A sternocleidomastoid tumour is an uncommon cause of a neck lump in neonates.

Pathology A sternocleidomastoid tumour is not a neoplasm; rather, it is an area of the sternocleidomastoid muscle that has become fibrotic and condensed.

Hypothyroidism	Hyperthyroidism
Overweight	Underweight
Slow movements	Hyperactive, tremor
Slow pulse	Rapid pulse, arrhythmia
Slow relaxing reflexes	Hyper-reflexia
'Toad-like' facies	Exophthalmos, proptosis
Pallor	Flushed or sweaty palms

Table 11.3 Features of thyroid disease.

Clinical features Neonates may present with a lump in the neck that is related (fixed) to the sternocleidomastoid muscle. If the muscle is significantly shorted there may also be abnormal positioning of the neck (torticollis).

Lumps in the groin

The differential diagnosis for groin and testicular lumps is wide. Two important conditions are:

- inguinal hernia
- testicular torsion

Inguinal hernia

Inguinal hernia is a common condition that presents with unilateral or bilateral groin masses, most frequently in male infants. It is particularly common in premature infants.

Pathology Infantile inguinal hernias are always indirect and are caused by a patent processus vaginalis, which allows herniation through the deep inguinal ring. The hernia may intermittently contain various abdominal contents, including bowel.

Clinical features Inguinal hernias present with a unilateral or bilateral mass arising from the deep inguinal ring and extending a variable distance but potentially all the way into the scrotum. The hernia may be intermittently present and should be checked for reducibility. If it can be reduced, it will often reappear when the child coughs or cries.

It is important to differentiate hernias from testicular masses – the key difference is that it is possible to get above a testicular mass but not a hernia.

Testicular torsion

Any boy presenting with acute testicular pain should be treated as a surgical emergency, owing to the possibility of testicular torsion.

Pathology Testicular torsion occurs when the testicle rotates inside the scrotum, occluding the blood supply from the gonadal artery. This causes necrosis, which becomes irreversible after 6–8 hours – hence the importance of recognizing this early.

Clinical features Acute testicular and abdominal pain are the main features of testicular torsion. On examination, the testicle is tender and either sits high or is retracted in the scrotum. There may be a blue discoloration visible through the skin.

> ### Clinical insight
>
> Remember that testicular pathology may present as abdominal pain in a young boy.

The main differential diagnosis is epididymo-orchitis, which can present in an almost identical way. Other differential diagnoses for a testicular mass are outlined in **Table 11.4**.

11.2 Examination of lumps and bumps

Introduction

Before examining the patient, a good history needs to be taken to establish how the lump started. Consider asking the following questions:

- how long has the lump been there?
- did it start slowly or quickly?
- is it one lump or are there many of them?
- is it sore? itchy? bleeding?
- are there any associated systemic symptoms, e.g. fever, vomiting, cough?

Inguinal hernia
Hydrocoele
Varicocoele
Epididymitis or epididymo-orchitis
Testicular torsion
Torsion of the hydatid of Morgagni
Testicular tumour

Table 11.4 Causes of testicular lumps.

- is the child well or unwell?

When examining a lump the following format should be followed to ensure that all the characteristics of the lump are properly assessed:

1. general inspection
2. site
3. size
4. shape
5. overlying skin
6. temperature
7. pain
8. consistency
9. mobility
10. regional lymph nodes
11. any special tests

General inspection

Inspect the patient for any obvious systemic disease and to assess the number of lumps involved, e.g. a patient with neurofibromatosis may have multiple cutaneous neurofibromas. Inspect the skin for rashes. Look at the lump you are being asked to examine in detail before laying a hand on it.

Site

Describe the position of the lump on the body. if there are multiple lumps, describe their distribution.

Size

Assess the size of the lump, using a measuring tape if available.

Shape

Describe the shape of the lump. For example, it may be ovoid, elongated or craggy. Palpate the edge of the lump and describe this.

Overlying skin

Identify any abnormalities of the overlying skin. For example, erythema is often seen in infection. Note any previous surgical scars.

Temperature

Feel the lump to assess whether the temperature is raised in comparison with surrounding areas. If the lump is hot, then this is another sign of infection.

Pain

Carefully palpate the lump (while watching the child) to assess for tenderness. If palpation causes the child pain then palpate very gently or stop the examination.

Consistency

Palpate the lump to assess the consistency of the contents. It may be hard (e.g. a bony lump) or soft (e.g. a lipoma). Feel to see if it is fluctuant; if it is, this indicates that it is filled with fluid.

Mobility

Examine the relationship of the lump to the surrounding tissues:

- assess whether the lump moves with the skin or whether the skin moves freely over it
- assess whether the lump is fixed to the underlying structures

This information is important because a knowledge of which tissue layer the lump is in helps to narrow the differential diagnosis.

Regional lymph nodes

Examine the regional draining lymph nodes for any localised mass. If there is an infected mass, there may be a tracking lymphangitis and there may be reactive lymphadenopathy.

Special tests

There are a number of further tests that can be performed, although they are not considered routine. Their use depends on the characteristics of the lump in question:

- reducibility, important when assessing a hernia – the child should be asked to cough; the hernia will re-form if it has been reduced before the cough.

- auscultation – bowel sounds may be heard, particularly in a hernia; a bruit may be heard over vascular masses
- fluid thrill – a percussion wave may be felt in very large fluid-filled masses
- transilluminence – a torch light shone through the mass will cause the mass to illuminate throughout if it contains clear fluid; helpful in detecting infantile hydrocoeles
- pulsatility – seen in some vascular masses, e.g. arteriovenous malformations
- resonance, useful when assessing large masses – a solid or fluid-filled mass is dull to percussion, whereas a gas-filled mass (e.g. a large hernia of gas-filled bowel) is resonant

Thyroid examination

The examination of the thyroid gland deserves special mention here because it is important to examine the patient for the systemic signs of thyroid disease:

- general inspection
- hands
- face and eyes
- neck
- legs

General inspection

Assess whether the child looks well or unwell. Consider whether the child is wearing clothing that is appropriate for the weather; children with thyroid disease may feel abnormally hot or cold.

Hands

Look for signs of hyperthyroidism:

- feel the palms of the hands for sweating
- ask the child to put the hands out straight and examine them for a fine tremor
- feel the pulse for tachycardia or an irregular rhythm (atrial fibrillation)

Face and eyes

Look for signs of thyroid disease:

- inspect the face, looking particularly at the eyes; excess white from the sclera visible above or below the iris indicates exophthalmos
- check to see if the eyes protrude forward (proptosis); this is best seen by looking from behind and above the child

Neck

The neck should be examined as follows:

1. inspect the thyroid gland from the front, and note the site of any mass and the characteristics of any overlying skin
2. watch the child swallow a glass of water and see if any mass moves; any mass that is attached to the anterior midline structures – a thyroid or parathyroid mass – moves with swallowing
3. while still in front of the child, ask him or her to stick out the tongue; a midline lump that is attached to the base of the tongue – a thyroglossal cyst – moves up as the tongue is stuck out
4. palpate the thyroid gland – this is best done standing behind the child sitting on a chair, but make sure the child doesn't feel intimidated by this; the gland should be palpated and described in the same way as for a neck lump (see above); check that the gland moves with swallowing
5. palpate for lymph nodes in the anterior cervical chain (**Figure 11.2**) and posterior cervical chain (**Figure 11.3**), under the jaw, behind and in front of the ears and at the occiput
6. finally, assess for the Pemberton sign; while standing in front of the child ask him or her to raise both hands above the head and hold them there – If the thyroid is enlarged this manoeuvre will obstruct venous return from the head and the face will become suffused

Legs

Finally, examine the legs:

- look for erythema nodosum, since it may indicate the presence of other autoimmune diseases
- test the patellar reflexes for the characteristic slow relaxation that is present in hypothyroidism

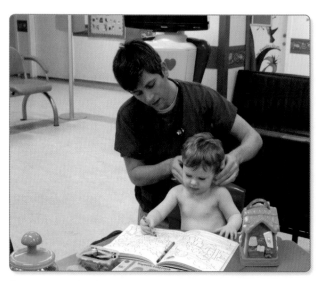

Figure 11.2 Feeling for lymph nodes in the anterior chain.

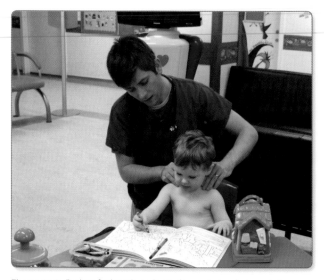

Figure 11.3 Feeling for lymph nodes in the posterior chain and above the clavicle.

| 'Jittery' or unsettled baby |
| Poor feeding |
| Tachycardia |
| Tachypnoea |
| Sweating |

Table 11.5 Features of neonatal hyperthyroidism.

Thyroid examination in the neonate

Newborn babies of mothers with hypothyroidism or hyperthyroidism may present with thyroid disorders in the first weeks after birth (**Table 11.5**). During pregnancy, maternal autoantibodies may cross the placenta and affect the developing thyroid tissue. This can cause a physiological surge in fetal thyroid stimulating hormone (TSH) at birth, and at-risk babies should have their thyroid function tests (TFTs) checked 5–7 days after birth.

It is important not to miss thyroid dyscrasia in the neonatal period because:

- hyperthyroidism may lead to cardiac failure
- hypothyroidism causes impaired brain development, which leads to the syndrome previously known as cretinism

11.3 Clinical scenario

A 4-year-old girl with neck lumps

A 4-year-old girl is brought to clinic after a GP referral – she has had persistent left-sided posterior cervical lymphadenopathy for the past 2 months. She initially had cough and cold symptoms, and a diagnosis of acute viral lymphadenopathy was made. However, she is now well, with no fevers and a good appetite. She has no past medical history. She is the eldest of three children and the family lives on a farm. She is fully immunised to date.

Initial differential diagnosis

Chronic lymphadenopathy localised to the neck can have a number of causes, the main ones being:

- postinfectious lymphadenopathy
- persistent infection, e.g. mycobacterial infection
- malignancy, e.g. leukaemia, lymphoma
- autoimmune disease, e.g. systemic lupus erythematosus

Further information

Examination demonstrates localised lymphadenopathy only: there are no enlarged lymph nodes in the axillae or groins, and there is no hepatosplenomegaly. The GP has performed a test for Epstein–Barr virus, which was negative, and has organised an ultrasound scan, which confirmed the presence of three enlarged lymph nodes in the neck.

Concluding differential diagnosis

The girl has a chronic localised lymphadenopathy, and it is therefore important to exclude malignancy as a potential cause. A referral to the ENT team for a biopsy is an appropriate next step.

Biopsy culture comes back initially negative, and histology is normal. A long-term culture shows a growth of a *Mycobacterium avium intracellulare* (MAI) spp., and surgical excision of the lymph nodes is curative. Follow-up immune investigations, including HIV testing, are all normal.

> **Clinical insight**
>
> Key points from this chapter:
> - there are important steps to follow when describing a lump
> - always consider systemic disease, even when the presentation is with a regional lump

Skin and rashes

Childhood rashes are very common, in particular viral exanthems and rashes from atopic diseases such as eczema. In addition, there are various congenital conditions that affect the skin.

The examination of the skin is an extremely important part of the overall clinical assessment, and it often gives clues to underlying systemic conditions – for example, café-au-lait spots are neurocutaneous markers that occur in neurofibromatosis. In acutely ill children, the skin may offer vital clues; a purpuric rash in meningococcal septicaemia is a classic example of this. Rashes in children can be extremely variable in their presentation. This chapter considers the common and important rashes rather than attempting to cover all skin lesions that may occur in children.

12.1 Common presentations

Erythematous maculopapular lesions

'Erythema' means redness, 'macules' are flat lesions, and 'papules' are raised lesions. Erythematous maculopapular rashes are therefore erythematous, the redness being due to inflammation, and they may be raised (papular), flat (macular) or a mixture of the two (maculopapular).

Key causes include:

- eczema
- viral exanthems such as measles
- Kawasaki disease
- erythema chronicum migrans

Eczema

Pathology Eczema is the commonest skin condition in children. There is inflammation of the structures of the skin. The cause is unknown, although eczema is strongly associated with other IgE-mediated atopic conditions, such as asthma, allergies and hay fever.

Clinical features The fundamental problem in eczema is skin dryness, which leads to the development of a scratch–itch cycle. This in turn leads to erythema, excoriation, bleeding and a risk of infection.

Treatment Treatment should consist of the use of emollients, bath oils and soap substitutes and the avoidance of triggers such as normal soaps, close fitting non-cotton clothes and (in some cases) dietary items. In inflammatory flares, corticosteroid ointment is needed. In cases of infection, antibiotics or antiviral medications will be needed (see Eczema herpeticum, below).

Measles

Pathology Measles is a systemic infection caused by a paramyxovirus. It remains one of the main causes of childhood mortality in the developing world. It is preventable with immunisation.

Clinical features The rash is said to start behind the ears and to spread down the body across the trunk and back (**Figure 12.1**). It is accompanied by high fevers. The child is miserable, with red conjunctivae. Early in the illness, Koplick spots (pale blue–white spots) can be seen inside the mouth next to the teeth.

Kawasaki disease

Pathology Kawasaki disease is a medium- and small-vessel vasculitis. The cause is unknown.

Clinical features and treatment The rash of Kawasaki disease (**Figure 12.2**) is non-specific, and diagnosis is made when the associated features are also present:
- red and swollen peripheries (**Figure 12.3**), with skin peeling
- fevers continuing for more than 5 days
- cervical lymphadenopathy
- bilateral non-purulent conjunctivitis
- redness or cracking of lips

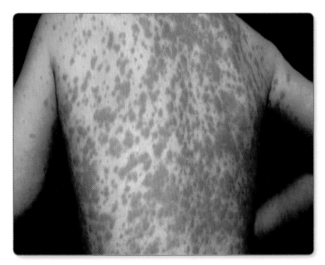

Figure 12.1 Measles.

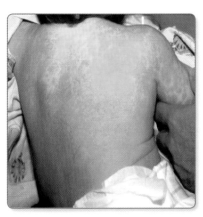

Figure 12.2 The rash in Kawasaki disease can be variable, and the other diagnostic criteria need to be considered before a diagnosis is made of Kawasaki disease is made.

Early diagnosis is crucial to prevent the potentially serious cardiac complications of Kawasaki disease, in which vascular inflammation may result in the formation of coronary arterial aneurysms.

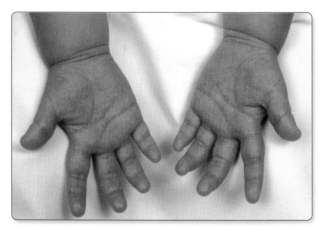

Figure 12.3 Swollen hands with a rash on the palms in Kawasaki disease.

Treatment involves the use of intravenous immunoglobulin and oral aspirin.

Erythema chronicum migrans

Pathology The target lesion in Lyme disease is erythema chronicum migrans. Lyme disease results from being bitten by a tick that is infected with *Borrelia burgdorferi*. The tick is found typically in woodland areas.

Clinical features Erythema chronicum migrans is a classic early manifestation of Lyme disease. It has a 'bull's eye' appearance (**Figure 12.4**).

Treatment should begin without any further investigation being needed, because serology for the infecting agent, *Borrelia burgdorferi*, is often negative in the early stages of the disease.

Vesicobullous lesions

Vesicobullous lesions are rashes in which the lesions are small blisters (vesicles) or larger blisters (bullae).

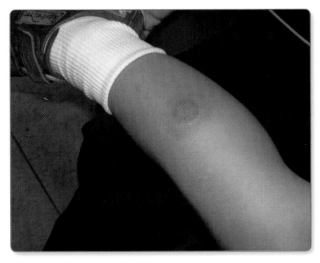

Figure 12.4 Target lesion of erythema chronicum migrans.

- Key causes include:
- varicella
- shingles
- eczema herpeticum
- bullous impetigo
- Stevens–Johnson syndrome

Varicella

Pathology Varicella (chickenpox) is the result of a systemic initial infection with the varicella zoster virus.

Clinical features A child with chickenpox has high fevers and may initially have coryzal symptoms. The rash develops as small, erythematous macules, usually starting on the trunk and back, then spreading down the limbs. The spots become vesicular (i.e. they form into small blisters), which then rupture and crust over. The rash may also involve the lips, tongue and tonsils, which makes drinking very painful.

Shingles

Pathology Shingles is a reactivation of varicella zoster virus. On initial infection with the virus, the widespread varicella rash is called chickenpox. The virus then lies dormant in the dorsal root and autonomic ganglia adjacent to the spine. The virus may reactivate at a later time. This reactivation may occur spontaneously or it may be due to a condition such as HIV infection that affects the immune system.

Clinical features The rash of shingles (**Figure 12.5**) has a classic dermatomal distribution, in that it appears across the area of skin innervated by one nerve root. Two or three adjacent dermatomes may be affected, and it may affect the face (innervated by CN V, the trigeminal nerve).

Eczema herpeticum

Pathology In eczema herpeticum, the thickened, dry and cracked skin of eczema becomes infected with herpes simplex virus (**Figure 12.6**).

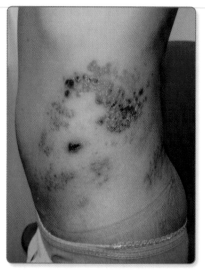

Figure 12.5 Shingles. Note the dermatomal pattern.

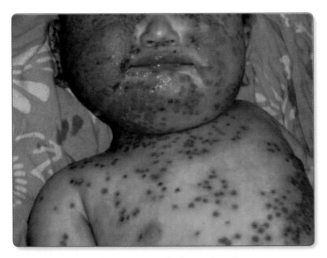

Figure 12.6 Eczema herpeticum on the face and trunk.

Clinical features and treatment The affected area of eczematous skin is markedly more inflamed and weeping than the other eczematous skin, and it is covered in small blisters.

It is important to recognise this condition – unless the area affected is very localised and the child is otherwise perfectly well, hospital admission for intravenous antiviral therapy (acyclovir) is indicated. In some cases, intravenous antibiotics are also required because of secondary staphylococcal infection (**Figure 12.7**).

Bullous impetigo

Pathology Impetigo is an infection of the dermis caused by *Staphylococcus aureus*. Fluid emanating from the infected site can raise a thin-roofed bulla or blister.

Clinical features and treatment Bullae with thin-walled roofs may rupture (**Figure 12.8**).

Intravenous antibiotics should be given, owing to the risk of rapid spread and systemic upset.

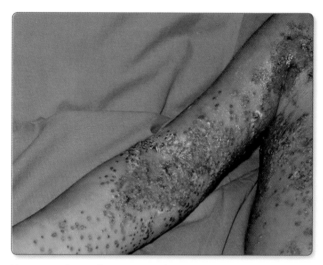

Figure 12.7 Eczema herpeticum on the arm. Note that some of the lesions have a golden appearance, which looks like impetigo and which suggests the presence of a staphylococcal infection as well as the herpes simplex virus infection.

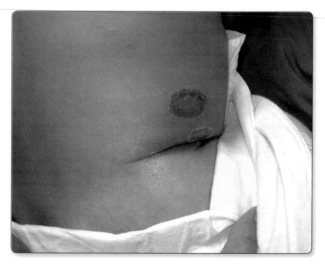

Figure 12.8 Bullous impetigo.

Stevens–Johnson syndrome

Pathology   Stevens–Johnson syndrome is a severe skin condition in which inflammation causes the epidermis and dermis to separate. It is usually the result of a drug reaction.

Clinical features   The clinical features form part of a spectrum; the severe form is toxic epidermal necrolysis.

There are bullae, with mucous membrane involvement (**Figure 12.9**).

Purpuric lesions

Purpura are small areas in which blood has extravasated into the skin. Pinprick-sized areas are called petechiae. Because the blood is outside the blood vessel, these lesions do not blanch on pressure (since the red blood cells are fixed in place).

The key causes are:

- Henoch–Schönlein purpura
- meningococcal septicaemia

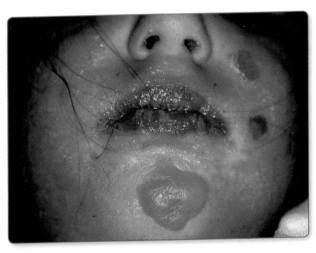

Figure 12.9 Stevens–Johnson syndrome.

Henoch–Schönlein purpura

Pathology Henoch–Schönlein purpura is a small-vessel vasculitis. The cause is unknown.

Clinical features The purpuric rash (**Figure 12.10**) occurs mostly over the anterior aspect of the legs, particularly the lower legs, and the buttocks. It may occur on the arms also. The main complications of the condition are:
- arthritis, usually affecting large joints such as the knees and ankles
- abdominal pain and, occasionally, intestinal bleeding
- intussusception
- acute glomerulonephritis

Meningococcal septicaemia

Pathology Bacterial infection of the bloodstream (septicaemia) results in inflammation of small capillary vessels. These vessels

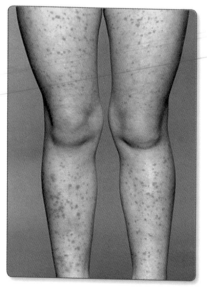

Figure 12.10 Henoch–Schönlein purpura.

become leaky, and red blood cells are able to extravasate into the skin and other organs.

Clinical features and treatment A child with meningococcal septicaemia is unwell. There may be fevers, tachycardia and hypotension, leading to impaired cerebrovascular perfusion and decreased consciousness. Small petechiae may initially develop and spread, extending in size and forming purpura.

Meningococcal septicaemia is a medical emergency, and the child requires intravenous fluid support and antibiotics.

Scaly lesions

In some conditions, a scale may form on top of a rash. Key causes of a scaly rash include:

- pityriasis rosea
- tinea versicolor
- tinea capitis
- psoriasis

Pityriasis rosea

Pathology The cause of pityriasis rosea is unknown, but it may be due to a viral infection.

Clinical features There is a 'Christmas tree' distribution to the rash (**Figure 12.11**). The rash is scaly, and it usually starts as a single area known as a herald patch, which is an oval, scaly patch. The herald patch is most commonly found on the trunk.

Tinea versicolor

Pathology Tinea versicolor is a fungal infection of the skin.

Clinical features In tinea versicolor, there are small circular areas of depigmentation. Even after treatment, the rash does not disappear until there is repigmentation following sun exposure. The rash typically affects the trunk, arms, axillae and back.

Tinea capitis

Pathology Tinea capitis is a fungal infection of the scalp.

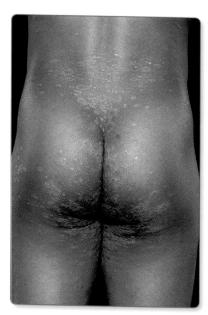

Figure 12.11 Pityriasis rosea.

Clinical features and treatment Tinea capitis may present as a localised area of hair loss or alopecia, with a scaly border. The condition is often misdiagnosed, particularly if a kerion is present (**Figure 12.12**), in which case it may be mistaken for an abscess. Scrapings should be taken for fungal culture from the edge of the lesion.

Topical treatment with an antifungal shampoo and systemic treatment with terbinafine should be started.

Psoriasis

Pathology Psoriasis is an inflammatory condition of the skin. The cause is unknown.

Clinical features In psoriasis, the skin is thickened and inflamed, with a silvery, scaly appearance. Psoriasis typically occurs in patches on extensor areas (the elbows and the knees); this is in contrast to eczema, which often occurs in flexor areas

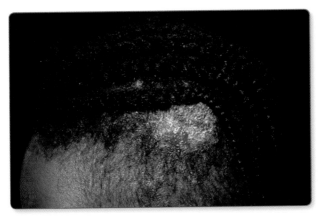

Figure 12.12 Tinea capitis causing a boggy swelling called a kerion.

(the antecubital fossae and the popliteal fossae). Psoriasis has systemic associations – in particular, there may be an associated arthritis. The nail beds may also be involved.

Urticarial lesions
Acute urticaria

Pathology Urticaria results from the degranulation of histamine by mast cells in the skin. The common causes are viral infection, allergy and drugs, but most cases are idiopathic.

Clinical features There is an erythematous maculopapular rash, with discreet raised circular lesions – the rash looks like the rash caused by stinging nettles (**Figure 12.13**). The rash does not cause scarring (often parents are concerned about this). Chronic urticaria is defined as lasting for longer than 6 weeks.

12.2 Examination of the skin

The key elements of the examination of the skin are a description of the general aspects of the skin, followed by a focus on the specific aspects of any lesions.

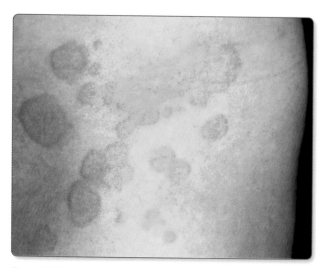

Figure 12.13 Acute urticaria.

General description

Consider whether the skin appears moist or dry. Skin that is dry and flaking may reflect dehydration, eczema or other, rarer conditions such as ichthyosis (literally 'fish-like'), in which the skin is scaly. Widespread peeling may reflect a recent infection such as scarlet fever, or a vasculitic illness such as Kawasaki disease.

Check for mucous membrane involvement, which may occur in toxic epidermal necrolysis and Steven–Johnsons syndrome.

Distribution of lesions

The distribution of any rash may give clues to the cause. A good example is Henoch–Schönlein purpura, in which the characteristic purpuric rash usually occurs over the extensor surfaces of the lower limbs, including the buttocks, but with sparing of the flexor surfaces. (Henoch–Schönlein purpura is a small-vessel vasculitis that affects the skin, gut mucosa and sometimes the renal vessels, and it can result in renal failure.)

Dermatomal

Some rashes occur in a dermatomal distribution, the most notable example being shingles (a reactivation of varicella zoster virus).

Scalp

Some rashes occur particularly in the scalp, the commonest of these being tinea capitis, a deep-seated fungal infection. Another way in which this condition may present is with a kerion.

Describing a rash

It is important to know the key terms used when describing a rash, and to have a structure whereby each property of the lesion or lesions may be described. Rashes and lesions should be described according to:

1. distribution
2. colour
3. shape and pattern
4. texture
5. contents

The nails, scalp and mucocutaneous junctions (the conjunctivae, nasal and oral mucosas and the perianal region) should also be examined (see Stevens–Johnson syndrome, below). Nail pathology can be the first sign of skin disease (e.g. pitting of the nails may herald the onset of psoriatic arthropathy).

Distribution

Describe whether the rash is:

- localised or generalised
- confluent or sparing of any particular areas such as glabrous skin

Colour

Consider the colour of any rash. A rash may be:

- white, indicating depigmentation – seen in tinea versicolor
- erythematous – seen with many inflammatory rashes and in eczema, measles and Kawasaki disease

- dark red or blue – seen in vasculitic conditions, such as Henoch–Schönlein purpura, and in congenital blood vessel malformations, such as a port-wine stain)
- brown – seen in skin lesions that arise from melanocytes, such as a giant congenital melanocytic naevus

Shape and pattern

Lesions may be described as being:

- round
- irregular at the edges
- linear or migrating (e.g. in shingles, cutaneous larva migrans)
- target lesions (e.g. in erythema multiforme, Lyme disease)

Texture

Lesions may be raised or flat, or a mixture of both. The skin surface changes may be indicative of a particular cause. Descriptions that are used to describe the texture of lesions include:

- macular – a flat, non-raised rash, seen in many acute viral exanthems
- papular – raised and palpable lesions, seen in acute urticaria
- scaly – seen in seborrhoeic dermatitis, psoriasis and pityriasis rosea
- crusty – most commonly occurs with exudates, such as seen in impetigo

Contents

Fluid-filled lesions may be:

- vesicular (< 10 mm in diameter) – seen in varicella zoster and herpes simplex (including eczema herpeticum)
- bullous (> 10 mm in diameter) – seen in bullous impetigo, Steven–Johnson syndrome and toxic epidermal necrolysis

12.3 Clinical scenario

A 3-year-old girl with a runny nose and red spots

A 3-year-old girl is sent home from nursery with a fever and runny nose. That evening, her mother notes that the girl is unwell and a bit lethargic, with a high temperature (40°C) and some red spots on her chest. Once the girl has had an antipyretic agent her fever comes down and she seems better. She is taken to see her GP the next day, when she again has a high fever.

Initial differential diagnosis

Fever and a runny nose alongside a rash suggest an infective cause, such as:

- measles
- erythema infectiosum ('slapped cheek' disease or fifth disease)
- scarlet fever
- meningococcal septicaemia
- roseola infantum (sixth disease)
- chickenpox

Further information

The girl is febrile but looks well, and is playing with a toy while sitting on her mother's lap. The spots are small, red, oval-shaped and raised, and they are on the chest and back, with some beginning to appear on the arms and scalp. The spots easily blanch.

The girl is fully immunised against measles, and she does not have the red eyes or any rash on the face that are typical of measles. In erythema infectiosum, caused by a parvovirus, the cheeks are affected, with a bright red rash. In roseola infantum, the rash develops when the fever stops.

Scarlet fever is an immune-mediated rash associated with a streptococcal throat infection. The rash may be red, but it is often fine, confluent and raised (described as 'sandpaper-like' in nature). Meningococcal septicaemia must be considered in a child with a rash and fever, but here the spots are blanching and the child appears well.

On direct questioning, the girl's mother mentions that a few children at a birthday party last weekend have come down with chickenpox, and that her daughter has not previously had chickenpox.

Clinical insight

Key points from this chapter:

- skin conditions are very variable, and they may be associated with systemic disorders
- a lot of experience is needed to be confident in recognising the variations in skin conditions, and a good dermatologist is invaluable to a team of paediatricians
- you should be confident in describing rashes according to the features described in this chapter

Concluding differential diagnosis

The girl probably has chickenpox. The spots will spread down the arms and limbs, form small vesicles and then rupture. They are itchy. There will be high intermittent fevers for 3–4 days. Once all the spots have crusted over, the girl will no longer be infectious.

Ear, nose and throat

Infections of the middle ear and the throat are a major cause of morbidity in paediatrics. Although these infections are usually minor, they are extremely common: between the ages of 1 year and 4 years, a child can have up to five or six episodes of otitis media or tonsillitis each year. Many of these children will present to their GP or an emergency department.

13.1 Common presentations

Painful ear

Differential diagnosis

The differential diagnosis of a painful ear in a child includes:

- acute otitis media
- otitis externa
- mastoiditis
- otitis media with effusion

Acute otitis media

Pathology Acute otitis media is a viral or bacterial infection of the structures of the middle ear. The tympanic membrane is inflamed.

Clinical features Because the majority of children with sore ears are of preschool age, the commonest presenting complaints are fever and vomiting rather than any localising pain – in many cases the child is too young to know the name of the area that is sore, or to explain 'pain' to an adult.

Children may be 'off their food' (because it hurts to open the jaw) or they may fall more easily (as a consequence of dizziness caused by fluid in the middle ear).

Some children are at increased risk of ear infections (e.g. children with Down syndrome or ciliary dyskinesias).

Otitis externa

Pathology In otitis externa, there is inflammation of the pinna (the earlobe). Otitis externa may be associated with a preceding otitis media or with an underlying immune deficiency. The bacteria that cause otitis externa include *Pseudomonas* spp., and bacterial swabs should be taken before treatment is commenced.

Clinical features and treatment The pinna may appear swollen, red, oedematous and crusty. The ear canal may be swollen or closed altogether.

Treatment consists of antibiotics, together with topical corticosteroids for the inflammation.

Mastoiditis

Pathology Mastoiditis is a local osteomyelitis – an infection of the mastoid process, the bony prominence behind the ear where the sternomastoid muscle inserts into the skull. Mastoiditis is a serious complication of otitis media – infection in the skull may lead to meningitis or a venous thrombosis, e.g. cerebral sinus thrombosis.

Younger children do not get mastoiditis because the bone is not yet fully formed and does not contain the air cells in which the infection can sit.

Clinical features and treatment The first-sign of mastoiditis may be the ear on the affected side being pushed forwards by the inflammation behind it and so seeming to 'stick out' more. The mastoid process is tender and red.

Cross-sectional imaging (with computed tomography scanning) may be useful for confirming the diagnosis.

This condition requires intravenous antibiotics, and may require surgery.

Otitis media with effusion

Pathology In otitis media with effusion, there are thick secretions behind the ear drum but no acute infection. Another term that is used is chronic serous otitis media.

Clinical features The child with otitis media with effusion may develop hearing and speech problems, caused by a conductive hearing defect across the fluid-filled middle ear. Recurrent infections may also occur. Most cases settle spontaneously, but if hearing is affected, then grommets (small aerating tubes) may be inserted into the tympanic membranes.

Sore throat

Sore throat is the most common paediatric presentation. Fever may be the only early presenting sign.

Differential diagnosis

The differential diagnosis of sore throat includes:
- tonsillitis
- croup
- epiglottitis

Tonsillitis

Pathology Tonsillitis is an infection of the tonsillar bed. The infection may be viral or bacterial, although it is often difficult to distinguish between the two aetiologies.

Clinical features The hallmark symptoms of tonsillitis are:
- fever
- being 'off food' (because eating hurts)
- vomiting
- lethargy

The tonsils are red, with or without exudate or swelling (**Figure 13.1**). There may be secondary tender cervical lymphadenopathy.

There may also be associated symptoms, for example:
- cough or coryza (a runny nose) in viral upper respiratory tract infections
- skin rashes in other viral infections, such as glandular fever (caused by Epstein–Barr virus)
- red lips and tongue (strawberry tongue) in some bacterial infections, such as scarlet fever (caused by *Streptococcus pyogenes*)

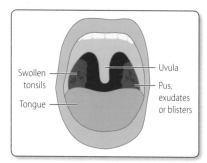

Figure 13.1 The appearance of tonsillitis.

Swollen tonsils

Tongue

Uvula

Pus, exudates or blisters

Croup

Pathology Croup is a viral infection of the larynx and trachea, usually caused by the parainfluenza virus.

Clinical features In croup, there is a characteristic cough with stridor. The throat is sore. (See Chapter 6.)

Epiglottitis

Pathology Epiglottitis is a bacterial infection of the epiglottis, usually by *Haemophilus* spp.

Clinical features The child with epiglottitis is unwell. There is drooling of saliva and stridor. (See Chapter 6.)

Epistaxis

Nosebleeds are a common presentation in the paediatric emergency department, and a few important points in the history should be checked.

Differential diagnosis

The differential diagnosis of epistaxis includes:
- mucosal trauma
- systemic coagulopathy
- a foreign body in the nose

Mucosal trauma

Pathology Any object that disrupts the thin, highly vascular nasal mucosa can cause bleeding. The most common such object is an exploratory fingernail. If a child has a cold or rhinitis, the mucosa can be thinned or swollen and therefore becomes more prone to bleeding.

Clinical features and management Nosebleeds are usually self-limiting. However, because the nose has a large blood supply (in order to warm inspired air), the amount of blood may look impressive.

Parents should encourage the child with a nosebleed to sit with the head held forward and to squeeze the soft tissue of the middle of the nose firmly until the bleeding stops. (Squeezing the bony bridge of the nose will not compress the blood vessels.)

Systemic coagulopathy

Pathology Bleeding may be prolonged in a child who has a condition in which there is a problem with the blood clotting cascade. Such conditions may be inherited (e.g. haemophilia) or acquired (e.g. leukaemia).

Clinical features Children with haemophilia usually have a family history of bleeding disorders, although up to a third of cases are *de novo* mutations. Acquired coagulopathies rarely present with a nosebleed as the sole symptom – there may be a history of lethargy, easy bruising, and bone or joint pain. If a child with a known coagulopathy presents with a nosebleed, a haematologist should be informed and local policies followed.

Foreign body in the nose

Pathology A foreign body in the nose can cause mucosal trauma. It is a common occurrence and the parents do not always know that it has happened. Children may put small objects (e.g. food, seeds, beads) into their nose and find that the objects do not come out.

Clinical features and management There may be no obvious sign that something is in the nose, or there may be a small amount of bleeding. If an object has been in the nose for a few days, offensive secretions may pass by it and be noticed by the parents – especially if it is an organic object decomposing in the nose.

Foreign bodies can be removed with a probe or suction. This may require a general anaesthetic if the object is firmly lodged (e.g. behind a nasal turbinate).

Another method of removing a foreign body is to occlude the unaffected nostril and ask the parent to seal his or her lips against the lips of the child and blow hard. This can cause the object to shoot out of the nostril, owing to the increased air pressure behind it.

13.2 ENT examination

Preparation is everything

It can be difficult to get a preschool child to co-operate for an ENT examination. The co-operation of a parent, carer or (with consent) another health professional is usually required. It is important to be firm yet kind. If a poor job is made of looking in a child's throat (e.g. if the child is inadequately held and is able to wriggle away), then the child will be even more distressed on the next occasion.

Check for cervical lymphadenopathy before approaching the ENT examination.

Ear examination

Positioning

Get the child to sit sideways across the parent's legs. The child's bottom should be on the parent's right thigh, with the child's left hip touching the parent's abdomen. The child should be sitting up straight, with the legs hanging over the left leg of the parent.

Ask the parent to wrap his or her right arm around the child's trunk and right arm, and to place his or her left hand on the child's forehead and temporal bone, above the right ear. This leaves the pinna of the child's right ear free to be held (see **Figure 13.2**).

Inspection

The following should be done:

- look at the pinna for any signs of otitis externa (inflammation, crusting or ooze from the skin)
- look behind the ear for a red spot of inflammation, which is suggestive of mastoiditis

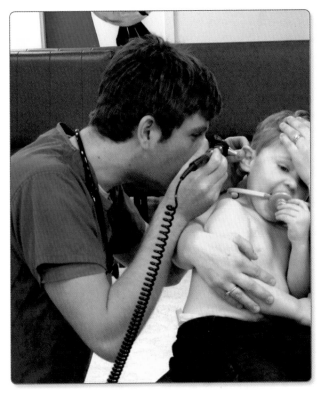

Figure 13.2 Holding a child for an ear examination.

- pull the ear gently backwards (towards the occiput) to straighten the ear canal, and look inside the canal; often the view of the ear drum is obscured by wax
- look for any pus or debris in the ear canal
- assess whether the drum is a healthy pink or is inflamed and red
- assess whether the light reflex (a reflection of light from the centre of the drum) is present; an absent light reflex is suggestive of fluid in the middle ear

Now turn the child the other way round and repeat the process to look in the other ear. If the process has been gentle and the parent is calm and reassuring, often the child will not struggle too much.

Nose examination

Positioning

In younger children the examination of the nose may be best performed initially with the child on the parent's lap. With a torch, observe the visible structures. Younger children are unlikely to tolerate the use of dilating instruments to aid visual inspection.

Inspection

Inspect the external structures and observe the mucosa overlying the nasal septum – the septum should be easily visible with a torch. There may be scratches on the mucosa if there has been any trauma (e.g. nose-picking leading to epistaxis).

It may be possible to inspect the nasal turbinates – the inferior and the medial turbinate may be visible. In allergic conditions such as rhinitis, the turbinates may be prominent, swollen or 'boggy' in appearance, and oedematous.

Throat examination

Because the throat examination is unpleasant, it should be the last part of an ENT examination in a child.

Positioning

With the child sitting up on the parent's lap (i.e. with the child's bottom pushed right back into the parents abdomen), ask the parent to place one arm across both the child's arms and to place the other arm across the child's forehead. Often children try to 'slip down' the front of the parent, so it is important that they are held upright initially.

Inspection

With a tongue depressor ready, ask the child to say 'aah'. When the child does this, quickly try to get the tongue depressor inside the mouth. Most children will then briefly gag, which, with a light held in your other hand and pointed at the throat, gives a good view of the tonsils and pharynx.

Unco-operative children will quickly snap their teeth shut on the wooden tongue depressor. Simply wait patiently; after a while they will open their mouth again to scream or cry, at which point it will be possible to depress the tongue and inspect the pharynx.

Inspect for inflamed tonsils, on which there may be:

- exudates (pus)
- multiple small sore vesicular blisters (in herpes simplex tonsillitis)

Look at the posterior wall of the pharynx, which may be inflamed in pharyngitis.

The roof of the mouth may have multiple small petechiae in infectious mononucleosis ('glandular fever'), which is caused by Ebstein–Barr virus infection.

Look inside the cheeks for Koplik spots, which may be seen in measles as small blue–white spots adjacent to the site where the cheek rubs the molar teeth.

There may be a foetor (bad breath) in tonsillitis.

If a throat swab (in cases of suspected scarlet fever) or a cheek swab (in cases of suspected mumps or measles) is to be taken, it should be done at this point. Have the swab ready in advance.

13.3 Clinical scenarios

A 4-year-old girl with a sore throat and a rash

A 4-year-old girl is brought to see the GP by her mother. The girl has been having fevers and has not eating much for the past 2 days.

Differential diagnosis

The differential diagnosis is wide because the presentation is non-specific. Fevers and being 'off food' is a common way for children to present.

Because of the fever, it is reasonable to start by thinking of infections, and what the likely site of any infection might be:

- otitis media
- tonsillitis
- pneumonia
- UTI

Further information

Today, the mother thought that her daughter's skin was 'rough' when she was dressing her. There has been no vomiting or diarrhea. The girl has no significant previous medical history and she is fully immunised. She has had a cough. There is no history of urinary symptoms.

The girl looks well and is sitting on her mother's knee. Her skin is not red, but it feels rough, like sandpaper, on her trunk, abdomen and back. Her breath is malodorous. There is no tachypnoea, and on auscultation the chest is clear. Ear examination is normal, but throat examination shows enlarged tonsils with bilateral exudates. A urine dipstick is negative for nitrites and has 1+ for leukocytes.

Concluding differential diagnosis and treatment

The girl has scarlet fever – group A streptococcal tonsillitis with a systemic rash driven by immune cross-reactivity. The treatment is 10 days of phenoxymethylpenicillin.

A 10-year-old boy with a sore ear

A 10-year-old boy comes to the emergency department with his school teacher. He has been complaining of ear pain for a day, and he vomited at school today after feeling dizzy.

Differential diagnosis

In an older child who is able to be specific about pain, the differential diagnosis is narrower than in a younger child:

- acute otitis media
- otitis externa
- mastoiditis

Further information

The boy has pus in his right ear canal, which prevents visualisation of the tympanic membrane. When the boy is observed from straight ahead, his ears do not look symmetrical: the right ear looks to be sticking out more. The skin behind the right ear is red and inflamed. When you pressing gently on this area, the boy cries out in pain.

> ## Clinical insight
>
> Key points from this chapter:
> - ENT examination is a core skill in paediatrics
> - be thorough – one good look in a well-immobilised child is better than multiple, ineffectual attempts

Concluding differential diagnosis and treatment

The boy has mastoiditis. He is referred to the ENT team, who organise a computed tomography (CT) scan. The scan confirms the diagnosis.

He is admitted for a course of intravenous antibiotics.

Eyes

Problems primarily involving the eye frequently present to paediatricians. The eye is also commonly involved in systemic diseases or central disorders, and eye problems may be the first clue of their presence (e.g. an intracranial tumour may present as an acute paralytic strabismus; see below).

14.1 Common presentations

The two most common presentations are a red eye and a lazy eye.

The red eye

The red eye may represent disease in the eye itself or disease around the eye with involvement of the surrounding tissues. Some of the common causes in childhood are:

- conjunctivitis
- preseptal cellulitis
- orbital cellulitis

Conjunctivitis

Conjunctivitis is a very common condition, which is seen particularly in younger children.

Pathology Conjunctivitis is inflammation of the conjunctiva. Many cases of conjunctivitis are due to viral infections (commonly adenovirus), but bacterial conjunctivitis is also quite common (e.g. staphylococcal infection). Conjunctivitis may also be an allergic phenomenon, commonly part of the symptoms of hay fever.

Neonates may have sticky yellow eyes that have an appearance similar to that of conjunctivitis but are more often due to incomplete canalization of the nasolacrimal duct. True neonatal conjunctivitis is due to infection acquired through the birth canal, usually with *Neisseria gonorrhoeae* or *Chlamydia trachomatis*.

Clinical features   Conjunctivitis presents with erythema of the conjunctivae, which may be seen best over the sclera. There is also often an exudate, which may be purulent in some cases (particularly in bacterial conjunctivitis). This exudate can cause 'sticky eyes', particularly in the mornings.

There should not be any reduction in visual acuity as a result of conjunctivitis – if there is reduced visual acuity, another cause should be sought, e.g. anterior uveitis, which can occur in connective tissue disorders.

Children with conjunctivitis may have symptoms of an upper respiratory tract infection or of allergy, depending on the cause of the conjunctivitis. Infective conjunctivitis is easily transmitted, particularly by children at school or in playgroups, and therefore it is important to ask about similar symptoms in friends or family members.

Preseptal cellulitis

Preseptal cellulitis is a common condition. It is also known as periorbital cellulitis.

Pathology   Preseptal cellulitis is inflammation of the tissues surrounding the eye, including the eyelids. It is caused by bacterial infection, most commonly by *Staphylococcus aureus*. Infection reaches the area by a number of mechanisms:

- local trauma
- local spread of bacteria (e.g. from sinusitis)
- haematogenous spread of bacteria

Clinical features   Children with preseptal cellulitis present with

- swelling
- erythema
- tenderness of the tissues surrounding the eye.

it may cause partial closure of the eye as a result of the oedema.

It is important that the features of orbital cellulitis (described below) should be excluded.

Orbital cellulitis

Orbital cellulitis is a relatively rare but serious condition. It can occur as a complication of the commoner preseptal cellulitis.

Pathology Orbital cellulitis is infection of the orbit, in particular the tissues behind the orbital septum (which differentiates this condition from preseptal cellulitis). The most common organisms implicated are *Staphylococcus aureus* and *Streptococcus* spp.

Clinical features Like preseptal cellulitis, orbital cellulitis can also present with erythema, swelling and tenderness of the tissues around the eye, but there may be some important additional features
- proptosis (anterior bulging of the eye)
- pain or limitation on movement of the eye, caused by inflammation of the extraocular muscles
- reduced visual acuity or loss of vision – a serious sign in orbital cellulitis

An urgent ophthalmology opinion is needed and the child will need intravenous antibiotics, a CT scan of the orbit and possibly surgery. Intracranial complications, e.g. cavernous sinus thrombosis, can occur.

The lazy eye

A lazy eye occurs where there is misalignment of the eyes, where one eye (the lazy eye) is not focused on the area where the child is looking. This can lead to permanent visual impairment (amblyopia) as the brain stops perceiving the image received from the lazy eye.

Two causes of lazy eye in a younger child are:
- strabismus (squint), which can be non-paralytic or paralytic
- cataract

Strabismus (squint)

Strabismus is a common finding in childhood; there can be varying degrees of squint ranging from a squint that is detectable only by a cover test (see below) to a squint that is obvious even to the untrained observer.

There are two forms of strabismus:
- non-paralytic strabismus, which is common
- paralytic strabismus, which is rare.

Pathology

Non-paralytic squint Non-paralytic squint is commonly found in children who have refractive errors; the squint helps them accommodate for these errors.

Paralytic squint In paralytic squint, a cranial nerve palsy affects the extraocular muscles, e.g. a CN VI (abducens nerve) palsy can cause a fixed convergent squint; such a palsy can occur in raised intracranial pressure caused by an intracranial tumour.

Clinical features The typical appearance of a squint is a misalignment of the eyes, with one eye appearing focused on the object in question while the other eye appears to be focused in a slightly different direction; sometimes the latter is called the lazy eye. In the common non-paralytic form of squint, the eye is able to move in all directions if formally tested; in the rare paralytic type, this is not the case and there is true paralysis.

Cataract

Cataract is uncommon in childhood; the commonest presentation is in neonates and infants.

Pathology A cataract is an opacification of the lens in the eye. Congenital cataract has a wide range of rare causes, including:

- intrauterine infection, e.g. rubella
- inherited cataract
- metabolic disorders, e.g. galactosaemia.

Clinical features The main finding is that of an absent red reflex on examination with an ophthalmoscope. There is also leukocoria (white pupil) on examination. Importantly, there is also likely to be reduced visual acuity on the affected side – this needs urgent attention in neonates and infants because reduced visual stimulation in one eye can lead to a permanent visual deficit (amblyopia). In severe cases the eye with the cataract may appear as a lazy eye if it is not receiving visual stimulus.

14.2 Examination of the eyes

The eye examination can be very brief, or it can be comprehensive, depending on the age of the child and the clinical situation. The steps outlined below should be followed to ensure a complete eye examination has been done, but various parts may be omitted in certain situations:

- general inspection
- examination of the structures around the eye
- examination of the front of the eye and fundoscopy
- assessment of eye function and neurological assessment
- cover test for strabismus

If there is concern about the clinical findings at any stage in the examination, or if an appropriate examination is unable to be performed, the patient should be referred to an ophthalmologist for slit lamp examination and ophthalmoscopy.

General inspection

Look at the patient:

- assess whether the child looks well or unwell
- assess whether the child is visually attentive, e.g. fixing and following on objects or faces; a neonate who is not fixing or following by 6 weeks of age requires urgent assessment – this can be a normal delay of visual maturation or a sign of eye or brain disease
- check for abnormal eye movements, e.g. nystagmus (a rhythmic jerking of the eye, which can be a sign of visual impairment or cerebellar disease)
- note any obvious strabismus
- look for any evidence of dysmorphism or signs of developmental delay, which may indicate diseases associated with specific visual disorders (e.g. refractive errors are very common in Down syndrome)

Around the eye

The following examinations should be carried out:

- assess the skin around the eye for erythema and swelling (indicative of preseptal or orbital cellulitis), and look for evidence of bleeding or bruising, which may be seen in trauma – consider child maltreatment

- examine the eyes for proptosis (anterior displacement of the eye in the orbit), which may be unilateral or bilateral
- examine the eyelids for swelling and erythema, and check for normal eyelid opening and for ptosis (drooping of the upper eyelid)

The front of the eye

Assess the following parts of the eye:

- the conjunctiva – look for redness and injection (as occurs in conjunctivitis); look for any discharge
- the sclera, which should be white in health – red sclerae may be due to scleritis or episcleritis, and blue sclerae may be seen osteogenesis imperfecta (brittle bone disease)
- the iris – look at the shape [an irregular iris may be due to posterior synechiae (scarring) as seen if there is a history of anterior uveitis]; look for any defect in the iris, which may be a coloboma (a congenital defect in the iris); look for blood or pus in the anterior chamber
- the lens – look for cataract (seen as opacification of the lens), which is best seen when trying to elicit the red reflex with an ophthalmoscope

Fundoscopy

An ophthalmoscope can be used to assess all parts of the eye, but it is particularly helpful for examining the retina. Fundoscopy is a difficult skill that is made more difficult by an uncooperative child.

First, ensure that the red reflex is present, by shining the ophthalmoscope into the eye and looking for the red reflection of the retina. Absence of the red reflex may suggest a cataract or a retinoblastoma. It is an extremely important clinical sign and must be acted upon immediately.

Clinical insight

A child who appears not to have a red reflex needs urgent assessment to exclude a retinoblastoma. This is often diagnosed incidentally when a family flash photograph reveals a lack of the red reflection in one of a child's eyes.

If there is concern about the possibility of raised intracranial pressure, examine the fundi and optic discs as would be done in an adult, looking for a blurred optic disc edge, which indicates papilloedema (**Figure 14.1**).

If there is suspicion of shaken baby syndrome, look for evidence of retinal haemorrhages, which can be associated with subdural haemorrhage and are therefore important to detect. However, detailed assessment of the retina in children is best done by an ophthalmologist using digital retinal photography.

Eye function and neurological assessment

To complete the eye examination, a full assessment of eye function is required. This is outlined in more detail in Chapter 9, but the steps below should be undertaken (if the child is old enough):

- pupillary reflexes to light should be tested and a relative afferent pupillary defect should be looked for

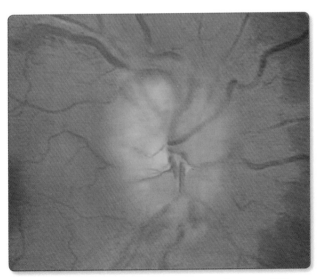

Figure 14.1 A swollen optic disc (papilloedema) seen on fundoscopy. With permission from Basak SK, Atlas on Clinical Ophthalmology. New Delhi: Jaypee Brothers Medical Publishers, 2006.

- visual fields should be tested, if possible
- visual acuity should be tested, using a Snellen chart if possible; in younger children, visual acuity should be texted crudely
- eye movements should be assessed by asking the child to follow an object while the parent holds the child's head still; this test is particularly important if there is concern over orbital cellulitis, which may cause painful eye movements

Cover test for strabismus

A child with strabismus (squint) has the eyes pointing in different directions while looking at an object (**Figure 14.2a**). This may be quite a subtle finding, but it can be seen on the cover test. Parents may notice the squint, particularly after taking a photograph of their child using flash photography, because the reflection of the flash will fall on different points in the pupils. This sign can be elicited in the clinic by shining a torch into the child's eyes and seeing where the reflections lie in the eyes. Strabismus is abnormal after 3 months of age.

To perform the cover test, sit immediately in front of the child and get the child to fix on an object. Then cover one of the child's eyes while watching the other eye. If the visual axis of the eye is correctly aligned, the eye will not move its gaze. If the eye is not correctly aligned, it will move to continue to focus onto the object (a non-paralytic squint; **Figure 14.2b**). If the eye is not correctly aligned but does not move (**Figure 14.2c**) then there is a paralytic squint (i.e. a problem in the central nervous system, a peripheral nerve or a muscle).

14.3 Clinical scenario

The clinical scenario below considers some of the concepts discussed in this chapter.

A 7-week-old boy whose parents are concerned about his vision

A 7-week-old male infant is referred by the GP because his parents are concerned that he is not seeing properly. He was

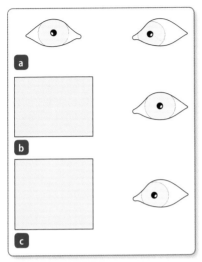

Figure 14.2 The cover test for strabismus. (a) Strabismus. The visual axis of the left eye is not correctly aligned. (b) The cover test. Here as the 'good' eye is covered (here, for example, with a square card), the left eye moves to take up the gaze on the object. This is a non-paralytic squint. (c) Here when the good eye is covered the left eye does not take up the gaze. This is a paralytic squint.

born at full term, without any concerns throughout pregnancy or delivery. He suffered from prolonged jaundice and has had frequent vomiting, and has not been gaining weight on formula milk.

Differential diagnosis

There are two main differentials for the boy's symptoms:

- visual impairment caused by an optic nerve or a central brain abnormality
- cataracts

Further information

On examination the boy is thin and still slightly jaundiced. There are no dysmorphic features and his head circumference is on the 50th centile for his age. He has a roving nystagmus of both eyes and there is no red reflex present in either eye. The neurological examination is normal. He has good head and truncal tone.

Concluding differential

The most likely diagnosis in this case is bilateral cataracts. There is no evidence of any developmental disorder, although he is still very young for this to be judged fully. Moreover, the combination of jaundice, poor weight gain and absent red reflexes strongly suggests this is a metabolic disorder, most likely galactosaemia. He requires blood and urine tests to check for this disorder, and a temporary switch to a lactose-free milk until the results are known.

> **Clinical insight**
>
> Key points from this chapter:
> - infection behind the orbit is an emergency
> - reduced vision in a neonate needs urgent referral
> - if unsure, ask and refer

Genetic disorders and syndromes

chapter

15

Inherited disorders tend to present in childhood and therefore they have historically been a large part of paediatric practice. Many disorders have an identified genetic defect, but many more as yet do not and the search for candidate genes continues.

Syndromes

A 'syndrome' is a recognised collection of features that, when occurring together in one patient, allows a diagnosis to be made that may give prognostic information and inform the parents' decisions about future pregnancies. Not all features of a syndrome have to be present for a diagnosis to be made.

Genetic tests

When a genetic disorder is suspected, there are a number of tests available to assess the patient's genome. Karyotyping is one of the more basic tests that assesses gross abnormalities of chromosomes, such as trisomy, in which there is an extra chromosome (as in Down syndrome). More advanced techniques include hybridisation using probes to identify regions of the genome. This can be done in a number of ways; one example is fluorescence *in situ* hybridization (FiSH) which can be used to detect chromosomal microdeletions (as in DiGeorge syndrome).

15.1 Common genetic syndromes

Three important genetic syndromes are:
- Down syndrome (trisomy 21)
- Turner syndrome (monosomy X, 45XO or mosaicism 46XX/45XO)
- DiGeorge syndrome (22q11.2 deletion)

Identifying a genetic cause for a syndrome is important, but the main focus for the paediatrician is providing care and support for the child and the family, in terms of:

- identifying and treating current problems
- predicting future problems
- providing appropriate referrals for information on future pregnancies
- organising support for the often complex needs of children affected with a syndromic diagnosis

Table 15.1 shows some other examples of commonly occurring or important syndromes a paediatrician is likely to encounter.

Down syndrome

Down syndrome is the commonest cause of learning disability and is one of the commonest genetic disorders. It affects approximately one child in 700.

Pathology

Down syndrome arises from excess copies of the genes on chromosome 21. 95% of cases are trisomy 21, in which there are three copies of chromosome 21 instead of the normal two. This occurs by non-disjunction during meiosis, creating one gamete (usually an ovum) with two copies of 21, giving trisomy when combined with a normal gamete. This is a chance event that

Syndrome	Genetic defect	Main features
Klinefelter	47 XXY	Male, tall stature, infertility, behavioural problems
Fragile X	X-linked trinucleotide repeat	Learning disability, large ears, macro-orchidism, behavioural problems
Noonan	Majority of cases: autosomal dominant inheritance of PTPN11 gene at 12q24.1	Pulmonary valve stenosis, webbing of the neck, short stature, bleeding tendency
Williams	7q microdeletion	'Elfin' facies, supravalvular aortic stenosis, learning disability
Angelman	Imprinting – inactivation of maternal 15	Happy demeanour, learning disability, microcephaly, seizures
Prader–Willi	Imprinting – loss of paternal 15q11-13	Hypotonia, developmental delay, learning disability, hyperphagia

Table 15.1 Common and important genetic syndromes.

increases in frequency as the mother gets older. For this reason, the probability of conceiving a fetus with Down syndrome rises with maternal age, from approximately 1:800 at age 30 years to 1:100 at age 40 years.

Clinical features

Down syndrome is associated with a characteristic appearance described in **Table 15.2**.

Associated conditions

Children with Down syndrome are at increased risk of a number of associated conditions (**Table 15.3**). These conditions should be included in a differential diagnosis when seeing a child with Down syndrome.

Multidisciplinary management

Children with Down syndrome may have complex problems from birth onwards, and involvement of a large team from many different disciplines is important. The role of the general or community paediatrician in such situations is to co-ordinate care from the other professionals.

Turner syndrome

Turner syndrome occurs in between one in 2000 and one in 5000 females.

General characteristics	Short stature Hypotonia Decreased intellect, with mild to moderate impairment (IQ 35–70)
Facial appearance	Brachycephaly (disproportionately wide head) Low set, rounded ears Flat nasal bridge Pronounced epicanthic fold Relative macroglossia (large tongue)
Hands	Clinodactyly (the fifth finger curving towards the fourth) Single transverse palmar crease

Table 15.2 Clinical features of Down syndrome.

Gastrointestinal malformations	Duodenal atresia Imperforate anus Hirschprung's disease (a segment of aganglionic bowel)
Congenital heart disease	AVSD (in 40% of patients) VSD (in 30% of patients)
Central nervous system	Epilepsy Alzheimer disease
Haematological malignancy	Acute myeloid leukemia
Endocrine system	Hypothyroidism
Others	Recurrent otitis media Lax ligaments and atlantoaxial instability Decreased fertility Strabismus

Table 15.3 Conditions associated with Down syndrome. AVSD, atrioventricular septal defect; VSD, ventricular septal defect.

Pathology

Turner syndrome (45XO) occurs where there is loss of one X chromosome in a person who is phenotypically female. It is estimated that 1% of all fertilisations *in utero* have a Turner genotype, but most of these fertilisations end in miscarriage and therefore the actual proportion of live births with Turner syndrome is much lower.

The external manifestations and phenotype are very variable and partly dependent on the genetics. Affected females who are mosaic (e.g. 46XX/45XO) often show a milder phenotype. In contrast to Down syndrome, advancing maternal age is not a risk factor for Turner syndrome.

Clinical features

The phenotype in Turner syndrome can range from simply having short stature and ovarian failure to having all the features of the syndrome (**Table 15.4**). Not all features need to be present for Turner syndrome to be diagnosed.

DiGeorge syndrome

DiGeorge syndrome is a relatively common genetic condition that affects approximately one in 2000 to one in 4000 people.

Pathology

DiGeorge syndrome is also known as 22q11.2 deletion syndrome; this refers to the region on the long arm of chromosome 22 that harbours the deletion that results in the phenotype of DiGeorge syndrome. This deletion affects the development of the third and fourth branchial pouches *in utero*, giving the clinical manifestations of the syndrome, as described below.

General	Short stature Lymphoedema of hands and feet, particularly pronounced at birth Gonadal dysgenesis (leading to amenorrhoea, infertility) Obesity
Learning difficulties	Visuospatial problems Mathematical difficulties Hyperactivity Poor concentration and impaired social skills
Facial	Low hairline Webbed neck Low-set ears
Chest	Broad (shield-shaped) chest Decreased breast development
Cardiac	Coarctation of the aorta Bicuspid aortic valve
Renal	Horseshoe kidney

Table 15.4 Clinical features of Turner syndrome.

Approximately 95% of cases of DiGeorge syndrome occur as a result of a *de novo* (i.e. newly arising) mutation, but in a small number of cases the syndrome is inherited from a parent in an autosomal-dominant fashion.

Clinical features

Key features of DiGeorge syndrome are shown in **Table 15.5**. The presentation of DiGeorge syndrome is so varied that it was previously split into a number of different conditions. Although these are now grouped into one syndrome, a variety of features may be present in one person.

15.2 Examination for genetic syndromes

Some children will have dysmorphism (unusual facial or bodily structural features) as their presenting problem. The paediatrician is responsible for investigating this presenting complaint and determining if a genetic syndrome is likely.

When examining a child who is dysmorphic and suspected of having a genetic syndrome it is important to describe all

Cardiac	ToF
	Interrupted aortic arch
	Truncus arteriosus
	VSD
Facial	Characteristic facies (long face, hypertelorism)
	Cleft palate and submucous cleft palate
	Velopharyngeal incompetence
Endocrine	Hypoparathyroidism causing hypocalcaemia, which can result in seizures in the neonate
Immunological	Immunodeficiency secondary to thymic aplasia or hypoplasia, giving a T-cell deficiency
Other	Learning disability and developmental delay
	Renal tract anomalies
	Hearing loss (both conductive and sensorineural)

Table 15.5 Clinical features of DiGeorge syndrome. ToF, Tetralogy of Fallot; VSD, ventricular septal defect.

findings carefully, rather than try to guess a diagnosis on first inspection. Follow the sequence:

1. general inspection, including height and weight
2. head
3. eyes
4. mouth, nose and philtrum
5. ears
6. chest
7. abdomen
8. limbs

Clinical insight

A detailed history is essential before carrying out an examination when a syndrome is suspected, particularly focusing on:

- antenatal history, including details of any antenatal screening
- problems in the perinatal period
- congenital anomalies detected at birth
- growth
- development and milestones
- family history

General inspection

Stand back and inspect the patient, looking particularly at:

- height and weight – many genetic disorders can affect growth, e.g. Klinefelter syndrome causes tall stature
- development and behavior – children with a syndrome that causes severe learning disability may be developmentally younger than their actual age

Head

Assess the size and shape of the head. In younger children check the sutures and fontanelles for closure. Genetic syndromes such as Russell–Silver syndrome can result in a triangle-shaped head that appears disproportionately large in relation to the body.

Eyes

The following should be examined:

- the palpebral fissures – do these slant upwards (e.g. in Down syndrome) or downwards (e.g. in Noonan syndrome)?
- the intercanthal distance – this may be increased in Edward syndrome
- irises – look for evidence of a coloboma, a defect in the iris

Mouth, nose and philtrum

Look at the shape of the mouth and the philtrum, which connects the mouth to the nose; a long thin philtrum is seen in fetal alcohol syndrome. Look for evidence of a cleft lip.

Look at the shape of the nose and the nostrils.

Examine inside the mouth to assess the teeth and look for defects such as a cleft palate, which is associated with many syndromes although it may be an isolated congenital abnormality.

Ears

Examine the size and shape of the ears; large ears may be seen in males with fragile X syndrome.

Assess whether the ears are normally positioned or whether they are low-set (as seen in Noonan syndrome, for example).

Chest

Look at the chest and assess the shape and size. Look for webbing of the neck into the chest (seen in Turner syndrome).

Cardiovascular examination

Complete a full cardiovascular examination (see Chapter 7) when considering a genetic syndrome, because many such syndromes are associated with congenital heart disease, particularly with valvular abnormalities.

Abdomen

Inspect the abdomen, and look at the patient from the back, since spinal abnormalities may occur in syndromes.

Examine the genitalia; look for evidence of an intersex condition (ambiguous genitalia). Assess testicular size, which may be increased (e.g. in fragile X syndrome) or decreased (e.g. in Klinefelter syndrome).

> **Clinical insight**
>
> Key points from this chapter:
> - know the features of some common genetic syndromes
> - have a structured approach to examination of a child who is dysmorphic
> - many professionals are involved with the management of complex disorders

Limbs

Examine the limbs, looking for any abnormal length (e.g. short limbs in achondroplasia) or any abnormal shape or positioning of the limbs (e.g. rocker-bottom feet seen in Edward syndrome).

Index

Note: Page numbers in **bold** or *italic* refer to tables or figures respectively.